THE HEART MAP FOR VITALITY

ADD MORE YEARS TO YOUR LIFE AND MORE LIFE TO YOUR YEARS

BY

ANIL GUPTA

ROYA MATTIS

ABBIE RICHIE

DR. RANDI RAYMOND

LOUISE LERMINIAUX, MBA

DR. RAVI K. RAHEJA, M.D.

JOHN BAXTER

DR. LEN LOPEZ

DR. MARYANN WOODS-OSIFO DC.

ALDO MANCINI

Table of Contents

Foreword by Anil Gupta

There comes a moment in life when we realize that vitality is not just about surviving another day—it is about feeling fully alive in every cell, every thought, and every breath.

This book, The Heart Map for Vitality, was born out of a calling to go deeper than symptom management. True vitality is not measured only in numbers like blood pressure, weight, or blood sugar. It is measured in energy, joy, purpose, love, and connection.

Each author in these pages has walked their own journey through challenges, breakthroughs, and deep insights. They bring you stories of resilience, practices of healing, and proven strategies that merge science and spirit. From the cellular level to the spiritual plane, from small daily acts of kindness to the profound wisdom of grounding, you will discover that vitality is not something outside of you—it is already within you, waiting to be awakened.

What makes this collection so powerful is the diversity of perspectives, medical doctors, healers, coaches, advocates, and visionaries, all uniting with one purpose: to help you reclaim your energy and step into a life of wholeness.

This book is not just information. It is transformation. It is your invitation to move beyond fatigue, stress, and disconnection into a state of radiant well-being. Allow these words to guide you into greater clarity, health, and light.

May you not only add years to your life but also add more life to your years.

With love,

Anil Gupta

The Love Doctor

Chapter 1

You Are Always Worthy By
Anil Gupta

T here is a story I often share in my coaching—simple, yet deeply powerful.

I hold up a $100 note and ask, "Who wants this?"

Every hand goes up.

"How much is it worth?"

Everyone shouts out one hundred dollars.
Then I crumple it in my hand, drop it on the floor, and grind it under my shoe.

"How much is it worth now?"

"One hundred dollars" say most of the people!
I pick it up—dirty, creased, and even more worn, and ask again,

"How much is it worth now?"

About half the people say one hundred dollars.

"Who still wants this?"
Every hand still goes up.

Why? Because its value hasn't changed!

The same is true for **you. You are the most valuable currency on the planet!**

No matter what you've gone through…

No matter what people say about you…

 The disappointments, the rejections, the moments you've fallen short… **your worth has never changed.**

No matter what – your value never diminishes.

But here's something even more important to remember:

Wherever that $100 note goes, whether it's in a wallet, a bank, a donation box, a restaurant, or a hospital, it brings value with it.

It can be used to feed someone, to bring healing, to create opportunity, to uplift or to buy anything. The $100 has the power to do that.

It doesn't matter how many times it changes hands—it **never stops serving.**
It **never stops adding value.**
It **never stops being valuable.**

It never loses any value!

You can spend that $100 in a store and that store can use that same $100 note to buy more goods and that same $100 note can then buy another $100 worth of goods, and it goes on and on. It is always serving, adding, uplifting, and creating possibility in every space it enters. It never stops giving value. It never gets tired or frustrated. It never beats itself up!

Think about that for a moment.

And neither do **you.**

Wherever **you** go, you bring value.

Think about that for a moment.

The day your parents found out you were going to be part of their famil brought great joy to so many.

The day you were born brought so much joy and love into the world. Everything you did was greeted with love and joy, you could do nothing wrong, You brought so much love into the world just by being you!

You bring so much value. Wherever or whatever you do. Whether you are in a room, with family or friends. In a business. In a relationship. In silence, in speech, in strength, in struggle. In your support, in your friendships, everywhere you go.

You are valuable, not because of what you do, but because of who you are.

You were valuable ever since the day your parents found out you would be blessing them with so much joy and love. Your brought so much love and joy before you were even born. And you continue to do so ever since!

Even if no one tells you. Even if you feel invisible. Even if you've made mistakes.
You still carry immense value.

Just like the $100 note, you are a currency of kindness, love, connection, joy and light in the world.

Why We Forget Our Worth

So many people walk through life forgetting this truth.

Why?

Because somewhere along the way, they were told they weren't enough.
Because they were judged.
Because someone made them feel like they had to earn love.
Because they were compared, criticized, or dismissed.

When you were a baby you could do nothing wrong you pooped you peed you broke stuff you messed things up and your parents would never get upset with you were the golden child there were lots of hugs and kisses and magical moments and fun things to do with plenty of time with the parents life was a joy it could not get any better. Whatever you did was accepted by your parents and you would get acknowledged, have wonderful words of encouragement, loved, have lots of attention, played with, fed, clothed, washed, everything was done for you happily and gleefully. There were no expectations.

Something happened. At some point, some expectations started to creep in. You had to tidy up, you had to clean up, you had chores to do, you had to feed yourself and you had to behave. Everything that you did wasn't met with love and joy, there were times where you may have been told off, scolded or not felt loved and wanted. Your parents had started having expectations of you.

As human beings we crave the love we once had as babies, so we had to come up with a way to receive love. We get feedback from our parents by our behavior, so when we do something that pleases them, we remember that and when we do something that displeases them we will also remember that too. So, we try and find something that pleases them and that can be relied upon in the future to please them and get their attention and love.

The sort of things that we do to get love and attention from our parents is -

Be very tidy/neat/clean/organized.

Be very obedient.

Get our homework done.

Get good grades.

Be athletic.

Be very polite/sociable/charismatic.

Be funny, comical, a jester or joker.

Be naughty because that brings us attention

Be studious clever smart intelligent.

Be an entrepreneur, musician, artist etc.

We always find a way. We may choose more than one way.

But let me offer you a powerful reframe:

> **Your worth was never meant to be earned.**
> **It was only meant to be owned.**

Reflection & Exercises: Embodying Your Worth

These exercises are designed to reconnect you to your unshakable value, deepen your self-awareness, and allow your worth to radiate from within. Set aside 10–20 minutes each day for these practices. Transformation doesn't require time, it requires **intention**, commitment, persistency and consistency.

How to Reclaim Your Worth

Here are some simple, powerful practices you can use right now:

1. *Write Yourself a Worthiness Letter*

Start with:
"Dear [Your Name], I want you to know that you are worthy because…"

Let it flow. Write from your heart. Don't second guess or doubt what comes up.
You'll be amazed what comes through.
Read it back to yourself on regular basis. Put a note in your calendar to remind you every day or every week.

2. *Anchor the Ripple Effect*

Purpose: Realize the invisible impact you've made on others.

Instructions:
Write answers to these prompts in your journal:

- Who has told me that I made a difference in their life?

- When did my presence bring peace, hope, or healing to someone?

- Where do I bring silent value that I often overlook?

- What would others say about me?

- Do I make people feel happier?

- Do I bring energy to the table?

- Do people like to listen to what I say?

Now, write:

"Even when I cannot see it, I know that my presence brings value."

You may not always *see* the value you bring—but it's always there.
People will always remember how you made them feel.
Your smile may have changed someone's day.
Your words may have lifted someone from the edge.
Your courage may have inspired someone silently watching.

You are a ripple of light in this world. Never doubt that.

3. **Mirror Work**

Look at yourself in the mirror each morning and say some powerful
self-healing and empowering incantations. I have examples below
Do it even when it feels awkward.

Especially when it feels awkward.
You speak them aloud with energy and intention, embodying the
emotion behind the words.
Let them flood your nervous system with truth. Just do them and
ignore any inner voices that will try and put you off or create doubt.

Say them standing tall. Take a deep breath. Energize yourself. Say
them with power. Say them like you mean it. Say them as if they are
the truth – and they are!!

- I am enough

- I am worthy of love and joy

- I make a difference

- I am a gift to this world

- I bring value everywhere I go

- I am resilient and unstoppable

- I am a source of love, wisdom, and strength

- I am deeply loved and supported

- I am healing, growing, and evolving

- I am seen, heard, and appreciated

- I matter

- I trust myself

- I am a powerful creator of my life

- I am divine, unique, and irreplaceable

- I am always bring value

- I am always valuable

- I don't need to prove my worth—just own it

- I am light. I am love. I am enough.

- I am strong

- I can handle this

- I always have

- I always will

- I am powerful

- I make a difference

- I am loved

- People love me

- I got this

- I am loyal

- I am gentle

- I am honest

- I am trustworthy

- I have great friends

- I am ready

- I am ready

- I am ready

- I love me

- I love me

- I love me

- I am ready bring it on

- I can handle this

- I always have

- I always will

- Today is the day

- I am free

- Free to choose

- I choose me

- I am worthy

- There is no past

- I make a difference

- I will create a new future

- Filled with love

- But first

- I must love me

- I love me

- I love me

- I love me

- When I speak people listen

- I am strong I'm powerful

- I can handle this

- I always have

- I always will

- I got this

- Today is freedom day

- I am free at last

- It's not about me

- It's about the difference I make

- I make a difference

- I make a big difference

- I'm ready

- I'm worthy

- I am truly worthy

THEN GIVE YOUR SELF A GREAT BIG LOVE HUG

- **Pro Tip:** Place a sticky note with these incantations on your mirror.

🌟 5. The $100 Note Visualization

Purpose: Connect emotionally to the metaphor.

Instructions:
Close your eyes and imagine yourself as a $100 note.

See yourself being picked up, passed along, used in stores, given to charity, deposited into a bank, gifted to someone in need, and received with gratitude. Bringing value wherever you go.

Making people happy with their purchases.

No matter how worn or crumpled you become, you are **still valuable**.

Take 5 slow, deep breaths and feel the truth of this in your heart.

When you open your eyes, say aloud:

"I bring value to every space I enter. I am priceless. I am worthy"

"I bring value to every space I enter. I am priceless. I am worthy"

"I bring value to every space I enter. I am priceless. I am worthy"

"I bring value to every space I enter. I am priceless. I am worthy"

Final Thoughts

You are not here by accident. You are here by design.

Your worth is not up for negotiation.
It is your birthright.

You are the $100 note—still valuable, still circulating, still creating impact.

Never stop giving. Never stop shining. Never stop remembering who you are.

You are not the dirt you've walked through.
You are the light that still shines despite it.

You are not your past.
You are your potential.

You are not a mistake.
You are a miracle.

Let the $100 note remind you:

No matter where you've been… what you've been through… or how crumpled life may have made you feel…

You still carry value.
You still make a difference.
You still matter.

Wherever you go – YOU bring immense value!

This is the Truth

THE TRUTH WILL SET YOU FREE

Celebrity Role Models of Worthiness

Oprah Winfrey – The Power of Worthiness

When we speak of worthiness, few public figures embody it as clearly as Oprah Winfrey. Born into poverty in rural Mississippi, facing abuse and systemic discrimination, Oprah had every reason to believe she wasn't "worthy" of success or love. Yet, she chose to see herself differently.

Her turning point came when she declared: *"You alone are enough. You have nothing to prove to anybody."* That belief became the compass of her life.

Worthiness Lesson: True worthiness is not arrogance, it's self-respect and inner knowing.

Health Connection: When Oprah stepped into her worth, she stopped punishing herself with food and began nourishing herself with love. Science shows low self-worth raises cortisol, weakens immunity, and fuels disease. A healthy sense of worth reduces stress, improves self-care, and protects overall well-being.

Reflection Exercise:

- Where are you waiting for others to validate your worth?

- How would your choices around food, rest, and relationships shift if you believed: *"I am worthy, simply because I exist"*?

Brené Brown – The Courage to Be Vulnerable

Brené Brown built her career by studying shame and vulnerability. But before she became a global voice, she struggled with perfectionism and fear of rejection. Her research revealed that people with strong worthiness beliefs live more connected, joyful, and healthier lives.

Worthiness Lesson: Vulnerability is not weakness, it is the courage to be seen as you are.

Health Connection: Perfectionism and shame fuel anxiety, burnout, and insomnia. Brené's worthiness practice of embracing imperfection led her to prioritize rest, boundaries, and mental peace, powerful tools for emotional health.

Reflection Exercise:

- Where are you hiding behind perfection?

- What would change if you allowed yourself to rest without guilt?

Lady Gaga – Born This Way

Lady Gaga has been open about her struggles with depression, PTSD, and fibromyalgia. For years, she tied her worth to her performances. But through therapy and self-compassion, she declared: *"You have to stop crying, and you have to go and kick some ass."*

Worthiness Lesson: Healing begins when we accept ourselves, quirks, struggles, and all.

Health Connection: Rejecting yourself fuels chronic stress and worsens illness. Gaga's self-acceptance helped her manage pain, reduce depression, and build resilience. Worthiness became part of her physical healing.

Reflection Exercise:

- What part of yourself have you been rejecting that deserves acceptance?

- How would radical self-acceptance impact your health today?

Dwayne "The Rock" Johnson – Strength in Struggles

Before becoming one of the world's highest-paid actors, The Rock battled depression and career failure. His breakthrough came when he realized his worth was not tied to external success, but to his identity as a resilient man of service.

Worthiness Lesson: Your value is not in your achievements, it is in who you are.

Health Connection: Once The Rock claimed his worth, he built a foundation of fitness, nutrition, and mental strength. Worthiness fueled the consistency that transformed his body and health.

Reflection Exercise:

- How could honoring your worth help you stay consistent in health habits?

- What would happen if you measured your value by your resilience, not your results?

Michelle Obama – Worthy of Voice and Health

When Michelle Obama became First Lady, she felt the weight of comparison and judgment. She asked herself: *"Am I enough?"* Her answer, *"Yes, I am"* — shaped her confidence and fueled initiatives like *Let's Move!*

Worthiness Lesson: Saying "I am enough" unlocks your ability to serve others.

Health Connection: Believing she was worthy of energy and vitality, Michelle prioritized exercise, nutrition, and balance. Her sense of worth rippled outward, inspiring millions to pursue healthier lifestyles.

Reflection Exercise:

- How might believing in your worth empower you to take ownership of your health?

- In what ways can your personal worthiness inspire and uplift others?

The Single Mother Who Chose Herself

- Maria worked two jobs to support her children and often neglected her own health. She told herself she didn't deserve rest or joy until her kids were grown. One day, she collapsed from exhaustion. In recovery, she realized her worth was not dependent on sacrifice. By honoring her worth, she began setting boundaries, eating better, and scheduling rest. Her children noticed and became healthier too.
- **Lesson:** Worthiness means recognizing that your needs matter too.
  Health Impact: Reduced stress, better sleep, and stronger family modeling.

The Retiree Who Found Purpose

- David retired after 40 years of work and felt "useless" without his job title. Depression and declining health followed. A turning point came when he volunteered at a local food bank and saw the difference he made. He realized his worth wasn't tied to a paycheck but to the love and service he gave.
- **Lesson:** Worthiness comes from contribution, not position. **Health Impact:** Improved mood, increased activity, and better heart health.

The Teen Who Said No to Peer Pressure

- Sophie was 15 when friends pressured her into drinking and skipping school. She struggled with self-esteem and wanted to belong. After attending a youth workshop, she chose to value herself enough to say *no*. That decision strengthened her confidence and kept her health intact during a vulnerable season.
- **Lesson:** Worthiness is the courage to choose your health over approval. **Health Impact:** Avoided risky behaviors, reduced anxiety, and built resilience.

The Patient Who Spoke Up

- James was battling a chronic illness and always accepted whatever his doctors said, even when treatments weren't working. Eventually, he claimed his worth by asking questions, seeking a second opinion, and becoming an active partner in his care. His health improved dramatically once he advocated for himself.
- **Lesson:** Worthiness means your voice deserves to be heard. **Health Impact:** Better treatment outcomes, reduced stress, and empowerment.

The Woman Who Left a Toxic Relationship

- Aisha stayed in an unhealthy relationship for years, believing she wasn't lovable on her own. After therapy, she recognized her worth and walked away. Choosing herself brought peace, better sleep, and the emotional space to meet people who truly valued her.
- **Lesson:** Worthiness is refusing to settle for less than respect and love.
  Health Impact: Lowered stress, improved mental health, and restored vitality.

To book Anil Gupta for speaking or coaching
https://meetanil.com/call

Website www.meetanil.com

For my Immediate Happiness best seller -
https://meetanil.com/happiness-book

Email Anil@meetanil.com

NOTES

NOTES

Chapter 2

Rise Again- A Tool for Leveraging Life's Challenges By Roya Mattis

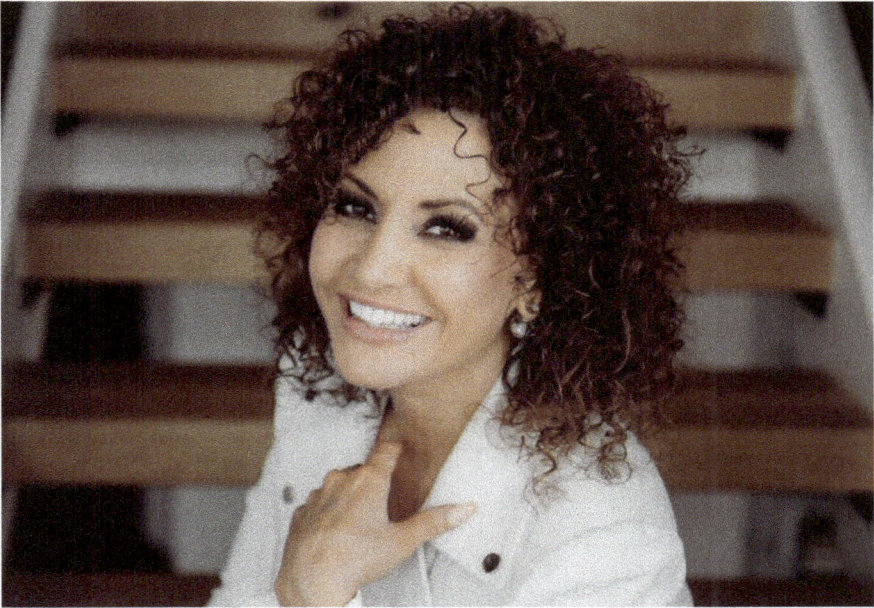

About the Author

Roya Mattis in her 25 year career mentoring entrepreneurs now focuses on creating deep lasting breakthroughs in the subconscious and in DNA passings via her **Creation of the *Trifecta Method™**. High impact leaders and public figures heal what no one else could reach - privately, efficiently, and permanently.

Roya is known for collapsing time to level up performance, profitability with deep purpose, relationship bliss, energy & peace. She is an Intuitive Healer and Certified Coach with Spiritual Gifts. Her approach is informed by countless hours of training to transform energy & deep wisdom into the fuel necessary to authentically up-level your life. Her trifecta of incorporating mind, body, and soul (with DNA reconfiguration) is efficient, efficient, and permanent.

Find out more at: www.royamattis.com

Rise Again: A Tool for Leveraging Life's Challenges By Roya Mattis

What if you're not trapped … you're just in a cycle? There's a rhythm to your life, a pulse beneath the noise. And yet, every now and again, what once seemed so certain starts to fray.

The relationship.

The energy.

The clarity.

The confidence.

Your body.

Your business.

Your voice.

You may be wondering, "What is wrong with me?" "Why can't I shake this?"

But what if it's not regression? What if it's a rebirth?

What if what you perceive as "the end" is actually the beginning of something deeper, wiser, and more in alignment with the person you are becoming?

You're in a Cycle, Not a Crisis.

In nature, nothing blooms forever. There's always a winter. Always a letting go. Yet we've been programmed to dread the shedding seasons. We fight against the release, judge the messiness as failure, and attempt to "push on through" via productivity.

But you can't "push" your way through winter and hope for summer.

That's why I am sharing this logical model of The Life Cycle of Change™: a simple, sacred framework that supports us in understanding where we are, what's happening, and how to rise through it.

The truth is: you're not stuck.

You are cycling. When you know where you are, you stop resisting, and you begin rising. I call this the Life Cycle of Change.

The instigator to your cycle is **Death: The Sacred Shedding**.

Each transformation starts with discomfort. A death, but not a real death. The moment it happens, it no longer fits like it once did. That might be something like a relationship, a belief, a version of yourself, or just a segment that once worked, but no longer does.

For me, one of my substantial "death" moments didn't occur at the bottom, but rather at a pinnacle of success: I reached the top 0.001% in my career and was leading thousands. Outside, I was "winning." Inside, I was dying. I remember a distinct moment after yet another 12-hour workday, realizing that I had begun a pattern of waiting for the familiar snore sound from the room next door, indicating that my husband was asleep. As I slid beneath the covers, I had a stark realization that this was my life, a life of avoidance. I didn't want it to be so. A new me was unearthing; a me exhausted by the life I had created. I was a corpse in my own life.

You may be in your Death Cycle. This does not signify a breakdown or that you're a failure. It means something is being invited to fall away. New growth in nature requires shedding. We are the same. This isn't the end. It's an invitation to make space for what's next. Too many are living as zombies. Their death cycles entrap them.

The first step out of Death is **Childlike Curiosity**. Just like an unfiltered child asking themselves, "What else can be true here"?

Once you allow yourself to let your mind wander about what may not fit for you anymore, there's a breath, a whisper. Something new is possible. Curiosity is invited. Begin asking questions out loud and to yourself. Pull back the curtain to other ways of being.

A significant time this stage showed up for me was when I found myself at a Tony Robbins self-improvement event. I couldn't put my finger on the layers of my silent suffering. I even felt guilty for 'suffering'. Addressing the audience, he asked: "If you're feminine at core, please stand up." I remained seated in my blinged-up heels and sparkly top, arms crossed, in total denial.

I was driving in my masculine 'doing energy'. Strategy, success, performance, that was my oxygen and my identity. But inside? I was tense, stressed, and felt the weight of the world on my shoulders as both an honor and a pressure. I had no 'safe place to be held'. Curiosity invited me to look at the parts of myself I had buried, in the name of efficiency, survival, and agreements to 'never be like this or that person''.

Things that once felt like enough were not anymore. What used to feel empowering to me, I had found, was now exhausting or frustrating me.

If you're in the Death Cycle, you're being invited. You're beginning to see again. Let it open you. Simply get curious. Attend the different things. Have the different conversations. Read the different books. Listen to different podcasts. Ask yourself, 'What else could be true here?'

Messy Adolescence comes next. Get ready. Just like adolescence is the entry point into becoming an adult, this part of the cycle is about you becoming the next version of you. And, like adolescence, it's uncomfortable. You try on new behaviors. You push boundaries. You overdo. You underdo. You feel exposed. Uncertain. Awkward. Here's where most people throw in the towel because this phase is confused as failure and can be truly uncomfortable. Hold on tight, friend, your breakthrough comes next! Do NOT recoil into the masses of the 'walking dead'.

I remember being willing to show up differently in my relationship and in life. Attempting to make boundaries, express emotions, alter the patterns, and explore this new femininity. My voice would shake. Sometimes I over-explained. Other times, I retreated. I even overdid it, too. It felt chaotic. But on the other side of all that mess was something stable. More authentic and less guarded.

I've witnessed this in clients over and over. One client, we'll call her Yvette, came to see me after 33 years of therapy. Additionally, she was a 2x Platinum Partner, which involved just under 1200+ hours of workshops over 2 years. She had tried everything, except this: root-level transformation. In one session with her, she moved from crippling social anxiety and insomnia to deep rest and peace. She slept through the night for the first time in years and was high-fiving strangers at a 1,500-person event that night.

You only get that kind of breakthrough in the mess. This phase is sacred. Stay with yourself. Have compassion for yourself. Imagine that awkward teen you can now have empathy for. AT LEAST you are ALIVE! LIVING! Out of the 'walking dead'.

Purposeful Adulthood: Anchoring in the new version of you. Finally, the fog begins to clear. You land on what feels true for you. You take direct action with purpose. The new habits, new beliefs, and new behaviors you've been trying are an anchor for the version of yourself that you are becoming. It takes decisive effort, but you have a map now! You are pressing play on what works.

It's not perfect, it's still tender, but it's anchored.

Hold fast to the routines, places, and people that are the essence of who you want to be next. Keep showing up for yourself. What once was hard becomes easy.

Maturity is Being. Maturity is embodiment, not perfection. It's integration.

It's when people call you the thing you've been becoming. When it's not something you do, but who you are.

Even now, it gives me pause to hear people say to me, "Roya, I just can't see you as this masculine-presenting version. You look and act like such a natural blend." I had to nurture that version of me. This is when I knew I had arrived at 'maturity'.

Linda is one of my most moving client stories. Linda was in a wheelchair when I started working with her. Diagnosed with M.S., she had weakened to the point of needing an extraordinary amount of energy to move her body any distance beyond a few feet. She was confined. Physically, Linda may have been considered to be in the 'Death Cycle'. Fortunately, her family took a chance and brought her to me.

We worked on all levels: the physical, the cognitive, and the ethereal. We started with the physical. The trust grew over time, and we gradually added the emotional and energetic. Something shifted.

Nine months later, Linda was walking 1.5 miles down the beach each day. She blows up rubber balloons to strengthen her lungs. She climbs entire flights of stairs.

She didn't just help heal her body. She regained her vitality!

That's Maturity. Not a finish line, an embodiment.

You no longer pursue the 'thing'. You become it.

Let's be clear, you can be in more than one cycle at the same time.

You might be in 'Maturity' in your career.

Messy Adolescence in your love life.

Death to your identity as a guardian.

Curiosity in your spiritual life.

It's not linear. It's layered.

Having an understanding that this process is natural is essential to authentic living.

When you realize where you actually are in each area, you stop beating yourself up.

Celebrate that YOU are AWAKE and MOVING through your journey. Not hiding from it like most people. You may also gain more compassion when witnessing others in their cycles, too.

You Were Never Broken. You are simply moving through the sacred, natural, wild, beautiful cycles of becoming.

It's how to transform from 'fixing yourself' to knowing yourself.

Now, thanks to the map of the Life Cycle of Change, you can rest in the understanding of where you are and what is next. Granting yourself even more permission to be alive rather than fear the cycles.

This is Your Season to Rise. Let go of the need to rush. There is no finish line. It's a sacred, spiraling journey back to yourself. You *will* rise again. Not as who you were and not as who you thought you would become. Instead, as the 'human becoming'. The one who walks through the fire, gathers your fallen ashes, and grows a garden out of them.

Let's Anchor This In. Which Life Cycle phase are you in in different aspects of your life right now? Write them down. Speak it aloud. Honor it.

And if you're feeling brave, share it with a friend. Once we give it a name, it becomes normal. And we make its liberation possible when we make it normal.

Conclusion: Along the journey of change, you'll discover even more that from ash (death) is fertile soil (life)! Every stumble, recovery, reinvention, ailment, fragility, collapse, has been a brushstroke in the artwork of this life, guiding you to your real work, soul work.

Want to Go Deeper? I can take you through practices and tools for each phase. Divine connection tools to go within for answers. Accessing your subconscious through your body. Uncovering the root causes of your DNA configuration influencing generational patterns. Most importantly, how to collapse time and go from surviving change to mastering change. You don't have to remain in the spiral. You are not here to shrink. You are here to RISE.

The Life Cycle of Change Recap

Curiosity. (Childhood) What else is possible?
Messiness. (Adolescence) Chaos and becoming.
Purpose. (Adulthood) Anchoring new truth.
Being. (Maturity) Peace and presence.
Shedding. (Death) Letting go. Making space.

These are not steps…they are spirals.
You are always becoming.
You are always allowed to begin again.

Let's Stay Connected

If something in these pages stirred your soul, I invite you to walk with me further.

Visit www.RoyaMattis.com to explore resources, courses, and ways to stay connected as you walk your own cycle of change.

Email Hello@RoyaMattis.com

Because transformation isn't a destination.

The life you dream of isn't waiting at the finish line.
It's waiting inside you—ready to rise from the ash.

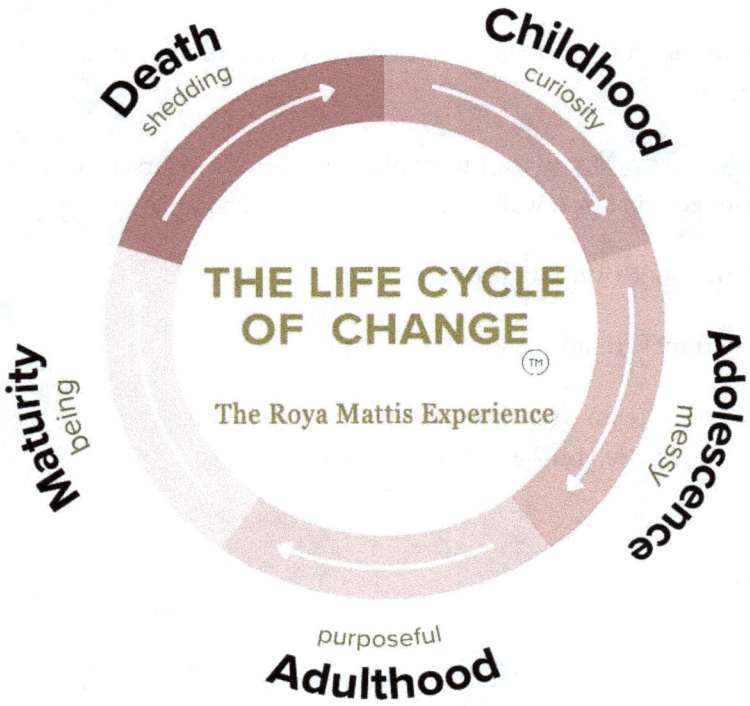

THE LIFE CYCLE
OF CHANGE
(TM)

The Roya Mattis Experience

Death shedding

Childhood curiosity

Adolescence messy

purposeful **Adulthood**

Maturity being

NOTES

NOTES

Chapter 3

The Tech-Savvy Path to Wellness By Abbie Richie

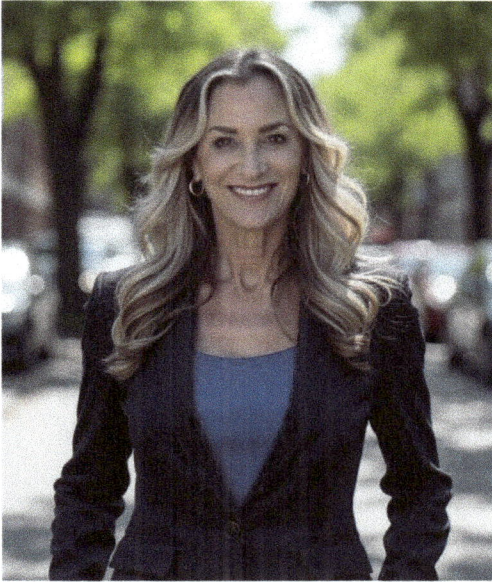

Abbie Richie is the Tech Guru at The Smarter Service. She is the host of Tech Smarter and Tech Talks on CBS Channel 3/5. Abbie is an experienced keynote speaker and has delivered presentations at TEDx, ICAA, AgeTechX Japan, LeadingAge, and AZ ALFA. She has been featured on The List TV, ABC, FOX, USA Today, AARP, and the Washington Post. You can reach out to her online at www.thesmarterservice.com and on social media, where she shares more tech tips via Instagram, Facebook, LinkedIn, and YouTube.

A lot happens in my car between 7:45 and 8:30 a.m. Taking my son to school has become something of a cherished ritual for me. Every morning, we listen to the Joel Osteen podcast, a routine we've happily maintained for five years now. Adam never complains about it; in fact, he often chimes in with his thoughts on Joel's uplifting messages. After I drop him off, I continue basking in Joel's profound yet straightforward insights for a bit longer.

But then, by 8:05, I circle back home to get my daughter, and just like that, the vibe changes. Faith's ready to take over the playlist, eager to blast her favorite songs on Spotify, DJing the ride to school as we belt out the tunes together. The tech in my car effortlessly aligns with my teens' individual needs, providing a soundtrack that resonates with their unique personalities.

Once I drop her off, however, I find myself craving a different kind of energy. I often switch off the music, embracing the silence that follows after all that transition. I limit the noise, podcasts, music, and news, and settle back into my rhythm without technology for those few precious moments before my workday starts. This practice not only feels refreshing; it is also a way to cultivate mindfulness and prepare myself for whatever lies ahead.

There is a balance and a method of allowing technology to enhance your wellness journey, without it becoming a distraction. Life is a wild ride, and as a tech guru, TV host, and mother of two diverse teens, I've learned how to blend the digital with the mindful, especially when it comes to personal wellness. Even in the hustle and bustle, it's possible to master tech while allowing ourselves the freedom to step away.

The Morning Ritual of Gratitude

Every morning, before school drop-offs, I start my day with a gratitude walk. It's simple yet profoundly grounding. I step outside, wearing a ridiculous, sombrero-sized sunhat, breathe in the crisp morning air, and walk - no AirPods, no phone, just me, nature, and my gratitude. This is my time to reflect, appreciate, and set my intentions for the day. As I power walk, I consciously think of all things I'm grateful for, mostly my kids, my loving family, and the fact that my parents are still alive. I love hearing the sound of birds chirping, smelling the starry white jasmine, and simply moving my strong body.

This daily practice has transformed my mindset, allowing me to start each day with a sense of purpose and joy. I don't care about tracking my steps or mapping my route; I immerse myself in the experience, truly tuning into my environment. And when you disconnect from technology for just a bit, it opens up a beautiful space for clarity and inspiration.

Finding Balance with Fitness Apps

Let's face it, technology can be a double-edged sword. On one hand, we have tools that make our lives easier, keep us connected, and help us pursue our wellness goals. On the other hand, it's all too easy to get sucked into a screen, scrolling endlessly through fitness stats or social media feeds. My approach? Use technology as your buddy. Master it, embrace it, and then give yourself the freedom to step away. You don't need to be with a friend 24/7, and you don't need to be constantly connected.

When I first started practicing yoga, I relied heavily on YouTube videos that would guide me through a class. I would create yoga playlists based on my preferences, whether I wanted to do flow or yin, and the time frame (sometimes I only have 20 minutes). I would have them all queued up and ready to go! But one morning, I faced a hiccup. The stinking video wouldn't load, and I was frustrated. "Grr! Hey, you! This is my zen time!" I had come to depend on its guidance, and that day, I felt lost without it.

In that moment of irritation, I took a deep breath. I calmed my racing mind and remembered the poses I had learned. I closed my eyes and connected with my body, leading myself through the sequences I had practiced so many times. As I transitioned from Downward Dog to Warrior II, I realized I didn't need the video prompts. I could rely on my knowledge, experience, and intuition. It was liberating to flow through the movements independently, finding my rhythm and reconnecting with my breath, just as the instructors always say you should do, right? That experience taught me that while technology can be helpful, the true essence of yoga lies within. It was a reminder that we often have everything we need right inside us.

Why? While YouTube offers fantastic yogi guidance, it's essential to reconnect with your body, your own awesome tool for wellness. Once you've learned the asanas and routines, try rolling out your mat without the app or video nagging you for your attention. Feel the stretch, the breath, and the flow of energy without the pesky notifications pinging in your ear. This is where you tune into your own wavelength, like a favorite song you've played countless times, yet every time, you hear something new.

My Disconnect and Reconnect with Health Tech

Ah, the Apple Watch, the technology staple that can feel like both a friend and a frenemy. It tracks your heart rate, reminds you to move, and lets you monitor your sleep patterns. So handy, right? However, there was a phase in my life when I relied on it so heavily that I began to feel defined by its data. Like when my heart rate would spike during a workout, and I'd get worried instead of enjoying the process.

One day, after a particularly frenetic week filled with deadlines and naughty teen drama, I decided to take a break. I left my pesky watch at home and went for a long walk around Lake Marguerite, a 20-acre lake in Scottsdale - yes, we have bodies of water in Arizona. Initially, it felt strange not to have that immediate feedback about my performance and the "what ifs" we parents constantly have. But as I continued, I noticed the rhythm of my breath, the simple joy of moving, and the freedom that came from not being tethered to technology. I rediscovered the pure joy of walking, not as a measure of achievement but as a celebration of movement.

And let me tell you, that experience transformed my relationship with my Apple Watch. I started wearing it less frequently, allowing myself to enjoy activities without the pressure of metrics. Going for a walk? Leave it behind. Instead, listen to the sound of your feet hitting the pavement and the rhythm of your breath. Tap into your intuition and understand what your body genuinely craves.

Embracing Mindful Meditation

We've all jumped on the meditation app bandwagon—who hasn't enjoyed a guided session while sipping coffee in their pajamas? Apps can be an excellent entry point to mindfulness. For a year, I was amazed at how calming it was to listen to Dr. Joe Dispenza guide me through my thoughts and feelings. But eventually, I realized my practice was evolving.

After a while, I became too reliant on technology for mindfulness. One day, I decided to put Dr. Joe aside and meditate without guidance. I closed my eyes, sitting cross-legged on my bedroom floor, with the sunlight filtering through the windows. The ambient sounds from the outside world filtered in, and I found myself listening to the rustling leaves and kids playing in the nearby park. It was as if I was tuning into a different frequency—a connection to both the moment and myself.

At first, my mind raced with thoughts: what was I going to wear that night, did I remember to send that important email, and why was I doing this anyway? It felt chaotic, but I reminded myself that it was all part of the process. Instead of forcing myself to silence those thoughts, I learned to acknowledge them and then gently redirect my focus to my breath. With each inhale, I felt a wave of calm wash over me, and with each exhale, I released any lingering tension.

This practice turned into a delightful experiment where I discovered not only how to breathe deeply but also how to simply be. It was the first time I understood what Dr. Joe meant when he said, "the space your body occupies in space." And trust me, this stumped me for a long time!

The beauty was in the simplicity, no guided voice (no hard feelings, Dr. Joe, I still love you), no chime telling me when to stop; just me and my breath. Slowly, I realized that while apps offer excellent guidance and structure, the essence of meditation lies in that personal connection to the self. I felt empowered to create my practice, using technology as a stepping stone rather than a crutch.

The Epiphany of Balance

As you gather insights from this journey, I hope you come to appreciate the gain and the joy found in disconnection. For me, striking that balance has been enlightening. The most meaningful experiences come from blending the best of both worlds: leveraging technology to support our paths to wellness while also allowing ourselves moments of sacred disconnect.

I often reflect on how we're surrounded by messages telling us that we need the latest app or gadget to stay healthy and fulfilled. But ultimately, the journey is inward. It speaks to the heart, toward knowing yourself beyond the data. It's about giving yourself permission to dance to your own rhythm.

Let me share one last personal story that encapsulates this. Recently, I attended a weekend wellness retreat where phones were discouraged. At first, I was all "grr" but soon felt released from the alerts, reminders, and data-driven life for those few precious days. The weekend became a mix of yoga, journaling, nature walks, and deep conversations with fellow attendees—all of us disconnected from our screens but profoundly connected to each other and ourselves.

During that retreat, I remember a deeper connection to my morning gratitude walks - I can take them anywhere I go, even when I visit my mom or I'm on a work trip. Then, the final evening, while watching the sunset, I found clarity like never before. I realized that the tech I often turned to wasn't a fit for wellness. Instead, it was my daily practices, like those quiet walks of gratitude and simple moments of presence.

Wrapping It Up

So, the next time you lace up those running shoes or roll out your yoga mat, take a moment to reflect. How can you embrace the tech you love while also finding freedom in disconnection? As you navigate this exciting journey, remember to allow yourself to experiment, breathe in, and just be.

Let's celebrate this beautiful balance between technology and simplicity and cheer for a wellness journey that's uniquely yours, whether it's morning gratitude walks, yoga sessions without an app, or meditations that tap into the depths of your soul, embrace your journey. Let it be filled with moments of mindfulness, reflection, and a sense of connection—both with yourself and the world around you.

Here's to mastering technology, harnessing its benefits, and then giving ourselves permission to step away and truly listen to our hearts.

NOTES

NOTES

Chapter 4

An Integrative Path to Wellness By
Dr. Randi Raymond

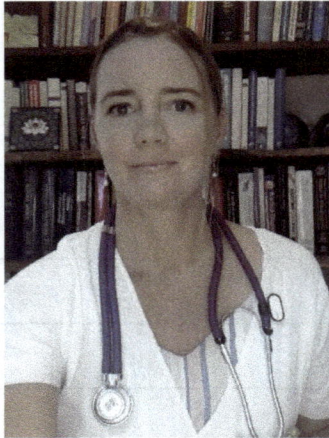

Combining ancient wisdom with modern technology to cultivate thriving health

As an integrative medical doctor, I combine Eastern and Western medicine to create custom wellness plans and experiences. I have more than 20 years of experience in health care and have always believed that the real answers for healing can be found in nature. I have lived in Costa Rica since 2003 and currently host one-on-one or small group wellness classes and experiences for guests from around the world at my wellness center Elev8 Health (www.elev8.health). I also lead health retreats at destinations around the world. I focus on Oriental medicine, farm-to-table nutrition, frequency medicine, cutting edge biologics, mycology, and plant medicine. My guests can also choose from other treatments including massage, colonics, ozone therapy, infrared therapy, yoga, meditation, qigong, life coaching, hydrotherapy and thermal therapy. I also own a plant medicine farm in Costa Rica that is adjacent to one of the most biodiverse, protected pre columbian rainforests in the world. I plan to build a research lab and expand my work with medicinal plants and mycology. I have created a space where you can be nurtured by nature and people who care to see you get healthy, thriving and back out on the playing field of life.

Over the past 20+ years of practicing medicine I have worked with thousands of patients and helped them through many life transitions. All of these experiences have shown me that there are many paths to wellness however there are many commonalities in our individual routes. I have been compiling the data over the years and have come up with an overall plan that can be followed by many who are looking to continue on their health journey.

Identifying the root cause of disease

So many of the people who find their way into my office have multiple vague symptoms that are difficult to pinpoint when and where they all started. It seems as dis-ease progresses it starts out mild so that we learn to adapt to it and then eventually there are multiple symptoms in multiple systems that begin to add up making normal daily tasks difficult. By the time we have reached this point it is very difficult for most practitioners to decipher what is the root cause so instead of addressing that they go after symptom management. It is unfortunate that western culture does not teach our children about self care, listening to your body, or trusting your intuition as those simple things would slow or stop so many diseases long before they could manifest into significant problems. The good news is there are some ancient techniques and modern tech that is making diagnosis of the root cause of disease so much easier. In all of my years of study and practice in eastern medicine I have found that understanding each person's constitution, current life cycle, listening to their symptoms, and taking a proper pulse and tongue analysis is a huge step in the direction of finding the root cause. When combined with modern DNA analysis, bio quantum scanning, magnetic resonance scanning, and WAVII brain scanning we are able to paint a complete picture of each person's current spot on their individual health journey. Once we have truly identified the root cause of their dis-ease it is much easier to begin to treat the underlying causes or deficiencies to help the body return to its optimal functioning levels.

Create your wellness plan

Once we have received your lab results we can identify the underlying and root causes of your dis-ease and begin to create a wellness plan to address your needs. Like anything, true health requires maintenance. That means we need to be aware of the thoughts we think, the food we eat, the people we surround ourselves with, and what we choose to do with our time. All of these areas need to be addressed and tended to on a daily basis if you want to create real change.

Detox and Cleanse

Next step is to implement your plan and get your health back on track. Options can include parasite cleanse, heavy metal detox, a liver flush, mold and yeast clearing, as well as viral and bacterial removal. Another option to consider is working with a de-prescribing pharmacist to reduce your medications and side effects by switching to more natural and effective alternatives.

Balance the systems

After detoxing and cleansing many systems of the body will begin to come back online. Now you can begin to focus on improving thyroid function, weight loss (if desired) with diet exercise and body protectant peptides, proper supplements, and bioidentical hormone replacement therapy. Acupuncture and herbal medicine can play a key role during this phase as this system has evolved over millennia to restore balance to the various systems of the body.

Mental Health

In the last couple of decades we have seen a sharp decline in mental health especially in western cultures. The focus on material wealth, poor nutrition, and isolation from loved ones has caused many to turn to medication to cope, In my opinion medicated depression is not a sustainable option as no one is suffering from a deficiency of zoloft nor do any of these antidepressant treatments address any of the root causes. If we are truly to resolve the mental health crisis we need to identify and treat any underlying vitamin or mineral deficiencies. We also need to address the core traumas that people have experienced and the best way I have found to do that is through the responsible and safe use of psychedelics, Either microdosing on a regular basis for a certain amount of time or macrodosing with a professional guide can be the profound shift that many need to help them change their perspectives and found a new route to happiness.

Continued self care routines

In order to maintain your health long term it is important to keep up with the maintenance. This can mean regular exercise, ice baths, saunas, supplements, acupuncture, massage, meditation, staying hydrated, good nutrition, gratitude, and following your joy. It takes only a few minutes a day to invest in your health in order to see huge gains in the long run. You are worth the effort and your attention to cultivating your personal health. At the end of the day you spend the most time with you so don't leave your wellbeing in the hands of others.

Reset the system

Once you have cleansed your body, improved your mental health, balanced your systems and created healthy routines you may be ready for a full system reset with stem cell treatment. This will improve overall health, and help retain long term benefits from all the work you have done. There are many options in this new and emerging field so do your research and choose wisely as to which therapeutic modality feels best for you.

Crafting your new life

Now that you reset your health you can continue on your new life path. Take the time to set goals for your next chapter and remember to do more of what brings you joy. No one has ever been at their deathbed and thought "I should have worked more" so please do yourself a favor and live every day with the end goal in mind. What do you want from this life to be happy and fulfilled? Don't be afraid to think about it, ask for it and enjoy it while it lasts. We only get so many trips around the sun on this rock we call home so let's enjoy and make the most of it.

Life routines to consider

People ask me all the time what I do for my own personal maintenance and so I thought I would write it down here to give you all a sneak peek into my routines and to maybe get some ideas of things you would like to implement into your life.

The number one thing I do is to do what brings me joy or puts a smile on my face as much as possible and ignore what doesn't. Also I try not to take things too seriously as I realize we never get "it" done so we can never get it wrong. What really gets me excited about life is the constant desire to create. Be it a great day or my next project. I enjoy being a creative force and continually watching things come together.

For health routines I guess I have to break them down into certain categories…. Things I do daily, weekly and once in a while.

Daily:

- First thing is rinse my mouth out to get rid of the bacteria from overnight

- Then face yoga and qi gong in bed while I listen to a gratuity meditation

- I drink one liter of water every morning with lime juice, ginger slices and a sprinkle of sea salt

- 5 minutes in the ice bath every day at 47' F

- 10-15 sun bathing after that to defrost and up my Vitamin D and testosterone levels

- Then I take my supplements....usually just NMN and a methylated multi vitamin. But occasionally I am experimenting with other things just to see how I feel. Sometimes shilajit, zeolite, seamoss, methylene blue, and mushroom extracts

- One cup of organic shade grown coffee per day with organic coconut oil and local honey. Ideally I drink this on my front porch watching the waves and the birds say good morning

- Then it's on to the "to-do" list of the day which includes farm chores that help keep me in shape

- For food I do my best to eat as seasonal, local and organic as possible. I avoid sugars and processed foods. I'm as farm to table as I can be. Other than that I prioritize enjoying my food, taking the time to savor and chew it, and I only eat with people I enjoy being around.

- I spend time with my kids, in my garden or with my animals everyday.

- At the end of the workday you can usually find me in a hammock enjoying the sunset with a glass of wine.

- After that it's usually a light dinner full of laughter and fun activities with people I love. Then I wind it down for the night time routine

- Sleep is a priority for me so I like to start slowing down around 8pm and preparing myself for bed with a relaxing shower or bath, then my skincare routine including castor oil with gua sha techniques and my tallow moisturizer. Normally I use some wild yam cream to promote my progesterone and boost my restful sleep. Then I read or watch a silly show and drift off to sleep.

Once a week I do use some NaD+ for the great boost in calm energy it gives me. I also do my best to have a self care Sunday where I spend the day doing body scrubs, mud baths, and whatever other hippy things I can think of.

Recently I received stem cells for the first time for longevity purposes. Based on my personal response and overall improvements to my health this is something I would like to continue once every other year if possible as the effects seem to last quite some time for me. I am also excited about the EBOO treatments as a way to deeply cleanse and reinvigorate my blood.

As technology is constantly evolving I am more excited now than ever to see what is coming next. I love researching and experimenting with myself and my own health journey so that I can improve my health and help those around me through my experience. As much as tech fascinates me I do have to acknowledge that the ancient activities of being with your tribe, farming, walking on the beach, cooking and following your joy are the real keys to happy longevity.

For more information you can find me at info@elev8.health www.elev8.health IG: CasaElev8

NOTES

NOTES

Chapter 5

Why Integrative Healthcare Matters: A Patient Perspective By Louise Lerminiaux, MBA

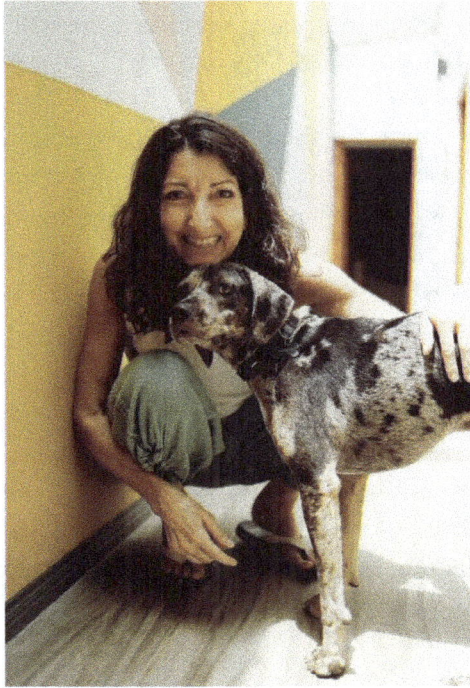

Louise has spent 30 years in program management in a variety of industries across Canada and the USA, with the last 14 years of her corporate career in life sciences and transplant diagnostics. Louise is the second generation of female transplant recipients in her family due to polycystic kidney disease. She received her unrelated living kidney at UC San Diego, California in Nov 2008 and was fortunate to avoid dialysis. She is a vocal advocate for patients to change the standard of healthcare based on her own personal transplant experience and her family members. Louise believes that a range of integrative medicine modalities

– western, eastern, holistic, regenerative, plant, spiritual - is what has enabled her to have a thriving life 17 years since her kidney transplant. Louise currently lives in Costa Rica with her intuitive Catahoula rescue Forest.

The term integrative medicine has many definitions depending if you are a western clinician, an eastern practitioner, a biotech scientist, a psychotherapist, a holistic healer, an insurance company, a pharmaceutical corporation, a caregiver or a patient. The definition has as many variations as the viewpoints you ask.

The challenge I encounter is the lack of collaboration to work together for the sake of the patient. Rather each perspective aims to persuade why their modality is better than the others. Humans are complex beings and because of this, we require a tapestry of care modalities to support our physical, mental, and spiritual health. As a Patient Advocate consultant, allow me to explain my experience.

I'm originally Canadian, grew up on a small prairie Catholic farm below the poverty line. Life was not easy on the farm. My father was a verbally and physically abusive alcoholic. I remember having uncontrollable eczema, severe allergies and annual strep throat my entire childhood. At age 5, my appendix was removed. It was the first of many hospital stays and surgeries.

I was often described as a shy or stoic child. I had learned early on if I kept quiet, I could avoid being yelled at or hit, and survive the living hell I was in. Reflecting back on it now, no one thought to ask what the cause of my eczema, strep throat and appendix bursting may be. If we had the financial means for therapy, I have no doubt I would have been diagnosed with complex post-traumatic stress disorder (C-PTSD) before I even started kindergarten.

At the age of 10, my mom had chronic kidney failure and needed dialysis. I remember being scared and wondering if she was going to die. Because we lived in a remote area, she had to take the bus into a city for dialysis, traveling 2-hours roundtrip, 3 times a week. With my 3 older siblings gone, I was forced into this adult caregiver role of both parents and my younger sister, even though I was just a child.

I left the farm at 17 and never looked back, unbeknownst to me, more traumatic experiences lay ahead. In my first year of university, I was date raped but too afraid to report it because in the 80's that wasn't done. In my 2nd year of university, I was diagnosed with the same genetic kidney disease as my mom, polycystic kidney disease (PKD). There was very little information. I had no idea if I would live to get married, have children, or see retirement. I would probably need a dialysis machine to keep me alive, or I would die before I got old. At 19, I thought 50 was old...I turned 58 this year, so I guess I'm old?!

But I was still alive, and there was enough time to start my career and I went for it. I worked in several industries, mostly in technical leadership roles. When I moved to the USA in 2002, I joined a global biotech. Having seen the medical impacts and gaps with my own care and that of my family, I wanted to work side by side with scientists to try to make a difference.

Meanwhile I kept searching for answers. In my late 20's, I started going to Adult Children of Alcoholics meetings, and reading every book I could get my hands on about the impacts of living with an addict. I began talk therapy to help me understand how the environment I grew up in wasn't normal. I began to practice yoga and studied Buddhism because the Catholicism I was raised in didn't align with my values. I started running marathons because it was a form of meditation and a way to stay healthy; though some would argue it was a form of addiction.

Then the reality of dying hit me like a brick when I was added to the deceased donor organ registry. I had less than 15% kidney function at the age of 39. So, what does that feel like? I was exhausted and freezing cold 24/7. I couldn't run, climbing the stairs to my bedroom left me winded. My eyes and skin began to yellow, food, even water, tasted like metal. My head was in a constant fog. My past endurance racing helped me muster up strength to go to work because I needed the income and medical benefits, but I would collapse into bed when I got home and sleep all weekend. I was told to write my will. What? I'm 39 and need to write a will? I was also scared about the medical bills because the USA healthcare system is very different. I debated moving back to Canada, but I was so sick, I decided to stay in San Diego.

When I was down to 10% in 2008, I was asked if there was anyone who might consider giving their kidney to me as a living donor. My best friend was the first to offer me her kidney and even though we were unrelated, we were a match. I will never forget that emotional phone call – it filled me with hope…and fear. You see, I've known her for over 35 years, and she always wanted to be a mom. She had had a premature baby a few months earlier so I told her no. I couldn't live with myself if she had complications and couldn't be a mom to her son. She assured me everything would be ok. She felt helpless when her son was in the intensive care unit for 1.5 months and this was her way to pay it forward.

It's still sometimes weird to think someone else's organ is inside of me keeping me alive. It remains to this day the most important lesson I learned in humility. I'm lucky because I now have 2 birthdays. My "re-birthday" is November 5 when my friend saved my life with her kidney. Later this year, it will be 17 years. I still feel some tiny relief when I hear the alarm in the morning knowing I am alive for another day. Living with an organ transplant is not easy and it's expensive. It requires a lot of specialists. I take daily anti-rejection pills that have nasty side effects like hand tremors, bone loss and bouts of cancer. I hate needles, but I can't avoid them. I had to give up dreams like crossing the Boston Marathon finish line, making it to Everest Base Camp or the hardest of them all, having my own children. But I honestly wouldn't change a thing.

While I am alive today because of the amazing western medicine advancements, I want this gift to last as long as possible. I want to be on the least number of pills, which tends to be the go-to solution in western medicine. It was apparent shortly after my transplant that I had to be responsible for my entire care. It was overwhelming navigating the complex USA healthcare system. I had to regularly see a general doctor, a nephrologist, a dermatologist, a gynecologist, plus an infectious disease expert.

I inherently knew I could not live with only that team. In 2009, I had my first myofascial massage and had immediate neuropathy relief in my legs due to scar tissue release from many abdominal surgeries. In 2011, I studied to be a personal trainer to help me understand this new body and offset the bone deterioration I experienced because of my medications. In 2014, I began acupuncture and experienced immediate healing benefits. In 2015, I started to study Japanese Reiki healing and eventually became a Karuna Holy Fire Reiki Master to help heal myself. In 2018 I got certified in Relaxation Yoga and Yoga Nidra to help with my blood pressure and ease the flight/fight world I still lived in.

I sought the help of my first naturopath in 2020 when one of my immune suppressant medications were causing HPV and cancer in my reproductive area. It was my first induction to the benefits of turkey tail mushrooms and herbs like curcumin to help reduce the cancer risks.

Talk therapy continued throughout the years off and on but it never really got to the core of numbness I felt. Hypnotherapy and Reiki helped a little but it wasn't enough. In recent years, my father then followed by one of my brothers both alcoholics died by suicide. I remember thinking "Great, another trauma experience to add to my already full complex PTSD diagnosis!".

By then I was a vocal advocate for transplantation and organ donation, but I was clueless on how to advocate for addiction and severe mental health diagnosis. I went through a Suicide Survivors program and learned about tapping, eye movement desensitization and reprocessing (EMDR) and mindfulness techniques that I incorporated.

After the Covid pandemic, I quit my corporate job and decided to move from Los Angeles and settle along Costa Rica's pacific coastline in 2022. The healing energy of its vibrant nature is palatable. I knew on my very first visit this is where I needed to be to deeply heal and more importantly thrive.

Shortly after I moved, I met Dr. Randi Raymond, the local integrative medical doctor. She was the first practitioner to spend 1.5 hours just talking to me. I did the Bioquantum Scan which highlighted many organ and mineral deficiencies. We started using the RIFE frequency machine, initially on skin issues and then specifically on the cysts on my native kidneys and liver. I resumed regular acupuncture and started slowly incorporating natural probiotics and teas.

I knew **Dr. Randi** (as she is lovingly known) also did clinical psilocybin treatments but I was scared and ill-informed. I volunteered at two clinician retreats to witness firsthand what their experiences were like. I saw these amazing shifts in these doctors so something told me I needed to pursue it.

We both were cautious so decided to start with a short dimethyltryptamine (DMT) session. The experience was profound – for most of it, I saw images of black sludge all across my abdominal and reproductive area. There was an outpouring and release of all this dark negative matter with a lot of bodily shaking. Towards the end of the session, these angelic beings flew in with silk banners and weaved my abdomen back together. I sobbed for a week after that, letting years of trauma be free while working with Dr. Randi to integrate the experience.

About 3 weeks later, I did another DMT session. This time my father was present and there was a lot of rage towards him that surfaced. There was a moment of seeing him as a child being abused and then it faded.

A level of forgiveness was felt. The most profound image was seeing myself in my 80's with long grey hair. I never believed, nor been told I could believe, I would live to an old age. For me, the image was telling me it was a possibility and was emotionally very liberating.

A month later, I did my first psilocybin treatment. I was intimidated because I knew it would be more emotional unlike DMT. I also felt it would open the decades of bottled up grief and sadness. I was scared once I started crying, I would not stop. The floodgates opened, with the initial hours all around my lost childhood. The experience transitioned to my organ transplant. The weight of responsibility to my friend to do everything possible to not screw it up. The expectation of receiving the gift unconditionally without feeling like I owed my friend anything. The utter exhaustion of the ongoing medical care and surgeries, something I had never expressed before for fear of seeming ungrateful. There was a lot of deep sadness and anger to acknowledge those feelings, which took months to process.

Since those initial sessions, I have continued with both psilocybin and DMT as layers of deep seeded trauma surface. I share these plant medicine experiences because I was a non-believer. I was terrified of doing anything to harm my transplanted kidney. Yet I also knew all the other modalities I had tried and incorporated over the years wasn't getting to the core of my brain to release myself from the numbness, and constant flight and fight mode.

In conjunction with these treatments, I was introduced to Family Constellations to heal generational trauma and illness. I participated in many sessions to examine my maternal and paternal patterns of trauma. The insights taught me how to release what no longer was mine, and extend forgiveness to my ancestral lineages. Somatic dance therapy also became a daily practice. Learning how to express emotions and reconnect with my mind and body in a free-form way has been liberating given my years of following prescriptive modalities.

One reality of living with an organ transplant is the daily immunosuppressant medication to prevent rejection are also toxic. A bit of a mind-fuck if I do say so myself. A few years ago, I was starting to see slow gradual declines in my kidney function. I was adamant I did not want dialysis or another transplant. I was committed to trying innovative modalities to prove there were effective alternatives. In the last year, I had the privilege of receiving mesenchymal stem cell and gene therapy infusions with the help and generosity of Mike Berkowitz and his team of experts.

From my years in biotech, I knew their effectiveness, but access was financially unattainable and still is for many people. We thoroughly and thoughtfully discussed options to help regenerate my transplanted kidney and regain function in my dormant PKD ones. While it is still early stages, I fundamentally believe we are going to prove this is possible. This can allow existing organ recipients the opportunity to extend their gifts of life, while permitting the limited supply of donated organs to go to someone new in need. Ideally I want to see stem cells and gene therapy be proactively used to avoid the need for organ failure treatment options in the first place.

As you can tell, I fundamentally believe in integrated medicine – western, eastern, holistic, spiritual, plant. There is no way I would be alive thriving in Costa Rica if I only followed western medicine practices. The next step is to remove the stigma and increase the cross-collaboration of modalities; while releasing the burden off the patient to figure this out on their own.

I didn't realize it, but integrative healthcare is what I have been piecemealing together since I left home 40 years ago. I know it's why I am still alive and why I feel my most important advocacy work is just getting started. Afterall, that 80 year old grey haired version of myself is counting on me and all of you to make her a reality.

Louise Lerminiaux, MBA

Patient Advocate Consultant

Wellness Consulting LRL LLC

Phone/WhatsApp: +1-619-876-2111 (CST)

Email: louise@wellnessconsultinglrl.com

Website: www.wellnessconsultinglrl.com

NOTES

NOTES

Chapter 6

Pre-Diabetes and Diabetes By
Dr. Ravi K. Raheja, M.D.

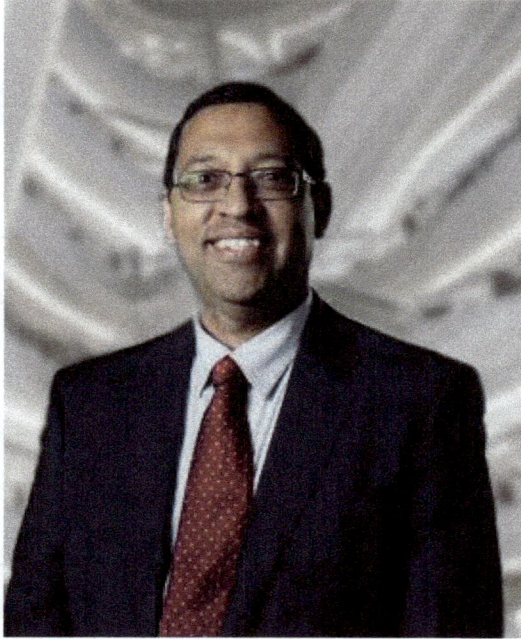

About the Author

Dr. Ravi K. Raheja, M.D.
Chief Technology Officer & Medical Director, TriageLogic

Dr. Ravi Raheja is a physician and healthcare technology innovator, co-founding and leading TriageLogic with the mission of making quality care accessible, efficient, and scalable. Trained at Robert Wood Johnson Medical School, he has built his career at the intersection of patient care and digital solutions, overseeing nurse triage programs, remote patient monitoring, and software that enables real-time insights—all designed to empower both providers and patients.

He has also developed platforms that allowed virtual nurse triage centers to operate seamlessly during recent healthcare crises, supporting systems like Baptist Hospital in Jacksonville. Through his role, he continues to bridge clinical expertise with technological innovation—turning ambitious ideas into tools that help prevent disease, improve outcomes, and reduce costs.

Prediabetes Explained

My Journey with Prediabetes

At 54 years old, I considered myself healthy. I exercised several times a week, ate what I thought was a relatively healthy diet, and always assumed I was at low risk for any kind of metabolic disease.

That's why what happened next came as a surprise.

When we released a new technology to scan and track vital signs, I began checking my numbers regularly. At first, my fasting blood sugars were in the normal range. Over the course of three months, though, I noticed they started creeping higher. At first, I dismissed it as a mistake in the readings.

But I decided to take it seriously and made an appointment with my doctor. Bloodwork confirmed what the scans had been showing I was prediabetic.

That moment was a turning point. Instead of ignoring the results, I made a commitment to change. I focused on my diet more carefully and planned to lose weight. Over the next six months, I lost 15 pounds. My fasting glucose levels normalized.

Today, I continue to monitor my health closely. I'm able to keep my blood sugars under control through lifestyle changes and regular vital checks—without medications.

For me, this experience underscored the importance of prevention, early detection, and taking action before a condition progresses.

Our goal is to educate people about how prediabetes and diabetes develop. Today, ninety-six million Americans live with prediabetes, and more than 80% of them have no idea their bodies are quietly struggling. That means millions are carrying an invisible condition that is already damaging their cells and organs — even though they may not feel sick.

By the time noticeable symptoms appear, the body has often been under strain for years. This "silent epidemic" is why awareness is the most powerful tool we have. If people recognize the warning signs and have access to simple, reliable tools for measuring blood sugar, they can take action before it progresses to type 2 diabetes.

"Prediabetes is not destiny — it's an invitation to act."

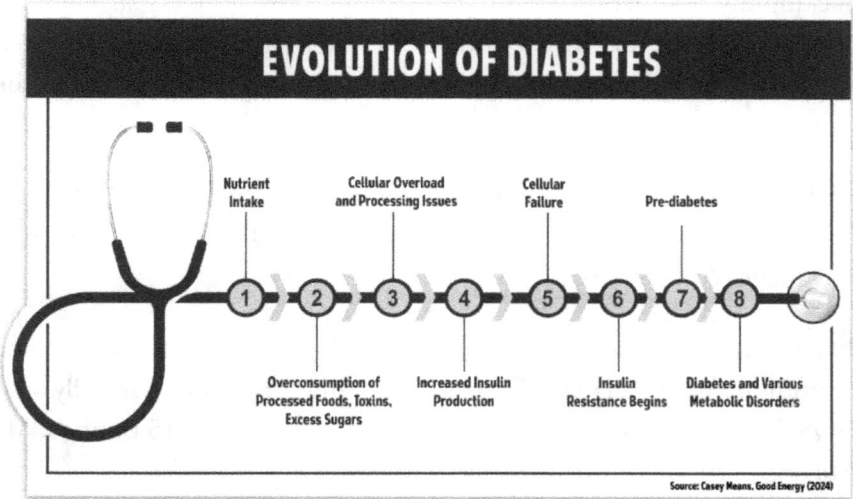

EVOLUTION OF DIABETES

Nutrient Intake (1)

Overconsumption of Processed Foods, Toxins, Excess Sugars (2)

Cellular Overload and Processing Issues (3)

Increased Insulin Production (4)

Cellular Failure (5)

Insulin Resistance Begins (6)

Pre-diabetes (7)

Diabetes and Various Metabolic Disorders (8)

Source: Casey Means, Good Energy (2024)

Understanding the Cellular "Factory"

The human body is made up of trillions of cells, each one a microscopic worker in a massive, coordinated factory. Their primary job is to take the food we eat and transform it into energy. When the system works, the factory hums along: nutrients arrive on time, waste is cleared away, and the machinery runs smoothly.

But like any factory, the system can be overloaded. When we regularly consume processed foods high in sugar, unhealthy fats, and additives, it's like sending wave after wave of delivery trucks to the factory gates. The workers can't keep up, the storage rooms overflow, and the extra shipments — glucose — pile up outside.

At the same time, harmful chemicals act like pollution in the factory. Toxins from pesticides, plastics, and even chronic stress corrode the machinery, making it harder for cells to function. The result is **metabolic stress**, a condition where the body struggles to process energy efficiently.

This stress builds slowly, often over years. That's why people may feel "normal" until suddenly a blood test reveals prediabetes.

The Role of Insulin: The Gatekeeper

Insulin is the body's master key. It unlocks the cell doors so glucose can enter. But with chronic overload, cells stop responding. This is **insulin resistance** — like workers ignoring shipments because the warehouse is already stuffed.

At first, the body compensates by producing more insulin. This "quick fix" works for a while, but eventually the signal breaks down. Glucose piles up in the bloodstream, leading to widespread damage.

"When the warehouse is full, workers stop accepting deliveries — this is insulin resistance."

Persistently high blood sugar inflames blood vessels, wears down the kidneys, injures nerves, and impairs the brain. It doesn't just increase the risk of diabetes — it raises the odds of heart disease, stroke, Alzheimer's, and more.

How to Break the Cycle

The hopeful truth is that this cycle can be interrupted. Studies show that people with prediabetes who adopt healthier habits can often restore normal blood sugar and avoid progression to diabetes.

- **Eat whole, unprocessed foods.** A balanced diet of vegetables, fruits, lean proteins, and healthy fats provides steady energy.

- **Limit sugar and refined carbs.** Avoiding sodas, sweets, and white flour reduces glucose spikes.

- **Move regularly.** Exercise increases insulin sensitivity and helps muscles use glucose more efficiently.

- **Reduce toxins.** Choosing whole foods, avoiding additives, and reducing plastic use lighten the load on your cells.

- **Sleep and manage stress.** Cortisol from stress and lack of sleep raises blood sugar — rest is vital for balance.

James Turns It Around

James, a 55-year-old accountant, was shocked when his doctor told him he had prediabetes. Instead of waiting for medication, he committed to walking 20 minutes after dinner and cutting soda. Three months later, his blood sugar dropped back into the normal range.

"Small, consistent steps are the strongest medicine."

Warning Signs of Trouble

Like a factory that starts breaking down, the body whispers before it shouts. Symptoms include:

- Constant fatigue

- Sugar cravings

- Brain fog or memory issues

- Belly weight gain

- Thirst and frequent urination

Many dismiss these as "just stress" or "getting older," which delays detection. That's why regular screening is essential.

Monitoring Glucose Levels: Catching Problems Early

Blood sugar testing is the most reliable way to know your risk. Common tests include:

- **Fasting Blood Sugar**: <100 mg/dL is normal; 100–125 mg/dL is prediabetes.

- **HbA1c**: Reflects 2–3 months of average glucose. 5.7–6.4% indicates prediabetes.

- **Post-Meal Glucose**: 140–199 mg/dL after two hours signals prediabetes.

- **Continuous Glucose Monitoring (CGM)**: A sensor worn on the skin that provides real-time patterns.

These tests give different perspectives. HbA1c reveals the long-term picture, while post-meal testing shows how food choices affect glucose in real time.

What To Do If Numbers Are High

Prediabetes isn't a guarantee of diabetes — it's a call to action. Simple shifts make a major difference:

- Cut sugary drinks and processed carbs.

- Add activity, even in short bursts.

- Experiment with intermittent fasting.

- Prioritize 7–9 hours of sleep.

- Track your glucose for feedback.

The Lopez Family's Choice

Both parents in the Lopez family were diagnosed with prediabetes. Instead of treating it as an individual issue, they made it a family project: cooking fresh meals together, walking in the evenings, and keeping devices off an hour before bed. Six months later, both parents had reversed their numbers, and their children learned healthier habits along the way.

The Bottom Line

Prediabetes costs individuals their health and the U.S. economy billions each year. According to the American Diabetes Association, the total cost of diagnosed diabetes is over **$327 billion annually**, including medical expenses and lost productivity. Much of this could be prevented through early detection.

How It Works

A new approach — **photoplethysmography (PPG)** — makes glucose testing more accessible. By shining light into the skin, a smartphone camera measures changes in blood flow. Algorithms interpret the signal to estimate glucose.

- **Accuracy:** 99.3% in identifying normal, prediabetic, or diabetic

- **Validation:** Clinically validate with thousands of data points

- **Accessibility:** Any modern smartphone with a flash can use it

"With just your phone, you can check your health — no needles required."

Looking Ahead

The implications are profound. By catching prediabetes early, we can prevent complications, extend healthy years, and reduce healthcare costs. Families gain peace of mind, communities lower chronic disease burdens, and health systems shift from crisis management to prevention.

Sarah's Peace of Mind

Sarah, a 38-year-old mother of two, had always worried about diabetes because it ran in her family. When she learned she could use her phone for quick checks, she felt empowered. When she noticed occasional spikes, she made adjustments to her meals and exercise right away. She also made an appointment with her doctor for further testing and recommendations. For her, knowledge wasn't just power — it was peace of mind.

Conclusion: Taking Charge of Your Health

Prediabetes is not a life sentence. It's a red flag that gives you time to act. By making lifestyle changes and using new technology, you can rewrite your health story.

A Gift for Your Health

As a reader of this chapter, I invite you to experience this breakthrough firsthand. You can access a free scan through your smartphone at ScanMyVitals.com/Vitality. With just your phone's camera and flash, you can measure your metabolic health — quickly, accurately, and without needles.

"Your health is not determined by fate — it is shaped by the choices you make today."

NOTES

NOTES

Chapter 7

Grounding to Frequencies By
John Baxter

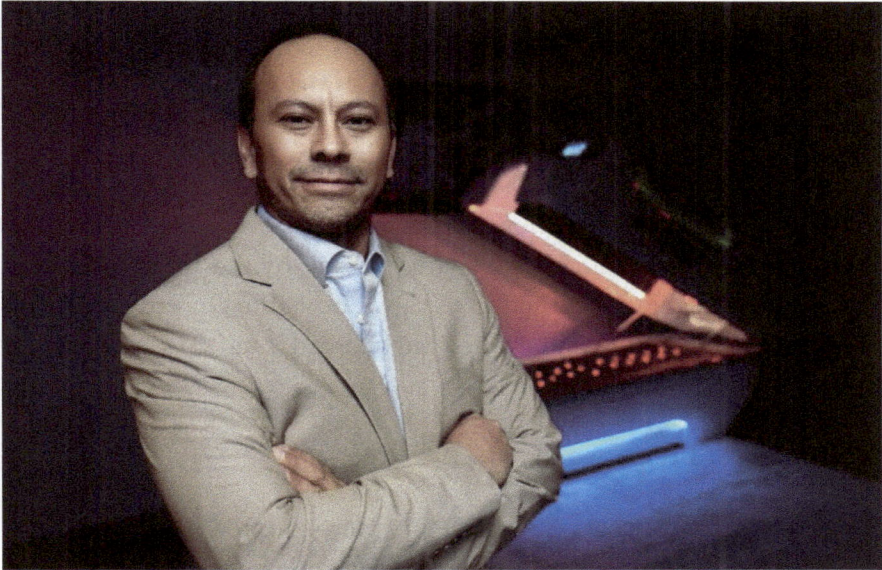

About the Author

Proven Innovator

With over 25 years in health and wellness, John Baxter has become a global pioneer in Med Bed Technology — merging biotech, anti-aging, grounding, frequency medicine, and biohackinginto a revolutionary new model of healthcare. As CEO of Anti-Aging Bed®, John has integrated more than 86 patented and proprietary technologies that are transforming the way the world heals, sleeps, and connects.

Massive Influence

John's message has reached tens of millions worldwide. His interviews on Charlie Ward's channel attracted an audience of over 20 million subscribers, with regular features on influential platforms such as Nicholas Veniamin's show, Superhuman Radio, and many more. His thought leadership spans across health, wellness, freedom, and technology — drawing both mainstream and independent media attention.

Recognized Leader

John was named Bloomberg's World's Greatest Health Technology Pioneer of 2024, solidifying his status as one of the most influential voices in wellness innovation. He was also spotlighted in a documentary narrated by Dennis Quaid, which highlighted him as the future of medicine and human longevity.

Champion of Free Speech

As the original producer of Patriot Party News, John created a platform that reached over one million views weekly with a strong commitment to free expression and independent thought. Today, he continues this mission through The Baxter Effect — fostering real conversations on politics, economy, frequency medicine, and the technologies reshaping our future.

Philanthropy & Purpose

John's companies have always carried a philanthropic mission at their core. He has donated over $4 million in Med Bed services and $1 million in products to those in need, while also spearheading Operation Honeybee, the largest "Save the Bees" nonprofit in the world. His vision is to align science, spirit, and service for humanity's highest good.

If I could give the world one message, it would be this: healing begins with grounding.

Everything I've ever built, everything I've engineered, everything I've lived through and discovered—has pointed back to this. Grounding is not a wellness trend. It's not optional. It is the single most critical component of the human healing system.

Without grounding, nothing works the way it should.

Without grounding, frequency medicine fails.

Without grounding, the body becomes a chaotic circuit—sparking, misfiring, miscommunicating.

The world today is drowning in frequency. We're blanketed in Wi-Fi, 5G, dirty electricity, satellite signals, Bluetooth pulses, high-voltage wiring, and invisible radiation that most people never even think about. Yet every cell in your body feels it. Every organ is impacted by it. Every night, when you try to rest, your body is trying to regulate itself while immersed in an invisible storm.

The truth is simple: you cannot heal when you're electrically overloaded.

This is where grounding becomes not just helpful—it becomes vital. Grounding discharges the buildup. It returns you to zero. It resets the field. And it's not just a concept—it's electrical law.

I've spent over two decades studying bioelectric medicine, inventing patented wellness technologies, and observing firsthand how the body responds to frequency. And here's what I learned: the body is not just biochemical—it's electric. Your heart is electric. Your brain is electric. Your nervous system is a network of signals, conductivity, voltage gradients. We are not made to run on static and chaos—we're made to run on coherence. Alignment. Earth's rhythm.

And that rhythm? That's the Schumann Resonance—a frequency emitted by the Earth itself, measured at roughly 7.83 Hz. That's not a coincidence. Our alpha brainwaves operate in the same range. This is not a spiritual metaphor. This is physics. We are designed to entrain with the planet.

When you stand barefoot on the ground, your body receives a flood of free electrons. These electrons are not symbolic—they are literal anti-inflammatory agents. They reduce oxidative stress. They neutralize the positive charges that accumulate from electromagnetic exposure. They bring your nervous system out of sympathetic fight-or-flight and into parasympathetic repair. In other words: grounding helps your body remember how to heal.

Let me say this as directly as possible:

The Earth is the original and ultimate healing frequency.

Every other frequency—whether it's light therapy, PEMF, sound medicine, Rife waves, Tesla coils, or scalar fields—must operate in harmony with that original signal. If the body is not grounded, you're delivering energy into a chaotic field. That's like playing symphonic music into a detuned radio. The message gets lost. The body can't decode it.

That's why every one of my technologies—especially the Anti-Aging Bed and Longevity Circuit—starts with grounding. Because grounding doesn't just help you feel better—it makes you receptive. It clears interference. It aligns the system. It turns your body into an antenna for healing, instead of a lightning rod for disease.

Now let's talk about what grounding really does—not just conceptually, but practically, biologically, spiritually, and electrically.

———

Grounding Electrically: The Physics of Discharge

The human body is conductive. You are 70% water with salts and minerals floating in solution. That makes you a biological battery—and batteries store charge.

Now imagine going through your day with rubber-soled shoes, synthetic clothing, and EMF-saturated environments. Your body builds up charge, but you have no outlet. You become electrostatically loaded. You're carrying unspent energy—and it manifests as tension, fatigue, anxiety, inflammation, even chronic disease.

Grounding acts like the ground wire in your house. It provides a direct, low-resistance path for excess charge to flow out. In other words: it bleeds off the voltage. That's not a poetic metaphor. That's measurable in real-time using voltmeters.

I've grounded thousands of people—literally—and every time we connect someone to our patented conductive sleep surface, their voltage drops from hundreds of millivolts to nearly zero in seconds. It's instant nervous system relief. The chaos is gone.

And the moment that happens? The body begins to receive the correct signals again.

———

Grounding Biologically: Anti-Inflammatory by Design

One of the greatest discoveries of grounding science is this: the Earth's electrons neutralize free radicals in the body.

Inflammation, at the cellular level, is an electrical imbalance. Free radicals are molecules missing electrons. They steal them from healthy tissue, creating a cascade of damage. But when you're grounded, the Earth acts as an electron donor—freely and abundantly.

Studies have shown that grounded subjects experience:

- Reduced C-reactive protein levels (inflammation markers)

- Lower cortisol

- Improved heart rate variability

- Thinner blood (reduced clot risk)

- Faster wound healing

- Better glucose control

- Reduced pain

All from simply reconnecting to the planet that made us.

———

Grounding Emotionally: The Nervous System's Home Base

We live in a sympathetic-dominant world. Fight. Flight. Phones buzzing. Traffic. Screens. Alerts. The sympathetic nervous system was designed for short bursts of survival, not continuous exposure.

When you ground, something shifts. You can feel it in minutes. Your breath slows. Your shoulders relax. Your heart rate normalizes. That's not placebo—that's the body exiting survival mode and re-entering its healing state.

Grounding calms the vagus nerve. It increases vagal tone. It literally helps you return to presence—because electrical coherence creates emotional coherence. You stop reacting. You start responding.

———

Grounding Spiritually: The Portal to Presence

This is the part no one talks about—but it may be the most important.

When you ground, you come back to the now. You stop being pulled into future anxieties or past regrets. You start to feel with your body. You sense energy. You remember who you are.

Many ancient cultures understood this instinctively. They prayed barefoot. They healed on the Earth. They slept on skins and dirt floors. We've "advanced" our way out of sanity and connection. Grounding restores the bridge between the human and the sacred. Between technology and nature. Between spirit and matter.

You begin to live in your body, not just in your mind.

And that is where the real medicine is found.

————

Grounding Technologically: My Life's Work

When I invented the Anti-Aging Bed, people thought I was just improving sleep. But what I was really doing was engineering a healing circuit.

Our grounding fabric—made with silver, carbon, and proprietary threading—connects the body to Earth potential every single night. No batteries. No devices. Just a clean, low-resistance path to reset the system. And unlike older grounding tech, which wore out after weeks, our system lasts for years—without loss of conductivity.

This matters, because grounding must be continuous. A few minutes a day is good. Eight hours a night is transformational.

Our technology allows frequency-based tools like PEMF and Rife to work with precision. Because the body is now tuned to receive.

Grounding Before Frequency: The Sequence That Heals

People always ask me: "Can I start frequency therapy right away?"

My answer is always the same: not until you're grounded.

If you deliver frequency into a charged, chaotic body, you may amplify the chaos. Frequency medicine only works when the field is clean. That's why every treatment, every upgrade, every activation protocol I teach starts with one simple commandment: discharge first.

This is the secret to unlocking the full power of the body.

Grounding before frequency means:

- You feel less fatigue during sessions

- You integrate frequency better

- You detox faster and with less symptoms

- You sleep deeper

- You become the tuning fork, not the interference

That's the future of medicine. Not pills. Not symptom suppression. But voltage. Frequency. Grounded precision.

———

Grounding Is the Foundation of All Healing

Let me say this clearly.

You cannot build health on an ungrounded system.

The most advanced tools in the world are useless if your electrical baseline is distorted. Whether it's medbeds, plasma therapy, scalar fields, or sound baths—none of it reaches the body properly if the "ground wire" is missing.

Grounding is not just step one. It's the platform. The chassis. The container that holds every other technology. It's the womb. The reset button. The truth.

It's how we come back to Earth.

It's how we remember who we are.

It's how we heal.

I didn't come to this through theory. I came through trial. Through pain. Through obsession. Through discovery. And now, I offer it to you— not just as a technology, but as a way of being.

Touch the Earth.

Sleep grounded.

Discharge your past.

Reset your field.

And become the frequency you were born to emit.

Because once you're grounded, you don't just absorb frequency—you become it.

And that's where the magic begins.

NOTES

NOTES

Chapter 8

Improve Your Habits and Attitude with 5 S.T.E.P.S. a Day by Dr. Len Lopez

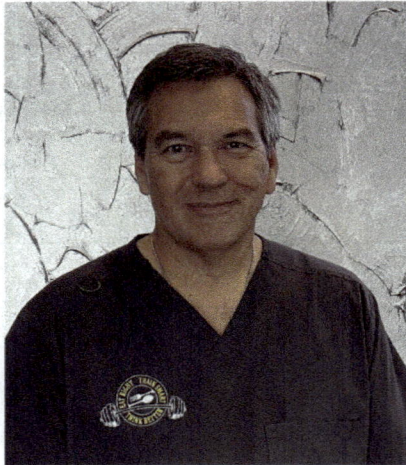

For over 25 years, Dr. Len Lopez has been using his background and training as a Clinical Nutritionist, Strength and Conditioning Coach, and Chiropractic Sports Physician to teach others how to Eat Right and Train Smart. His speaking skills allowed him to become the natural medicine expert for Good Morning Texas and Natural Health Made Simple. He stepped out of his comfort zone and started formulating nutritional products; invented My Portable Pullup Bar; and is now helping people Think and Dream Better with 5 STEPS a Day. To learn more visit www.DrLenOnline.com

For centuries, we've known 'you are what you eat and what you think.'

2,500 years ago, Hippocrates, the Father of Medicine said, "let food be your medicine and let medicine be your food." Way back then, in ancient times, he knew what you put into your body can make you healthy and strong, just as easily as it can make you weak and lethargic.

The Bible, Confucius, and Buddha said something similar with regards to the thoughts that feed your mind and said, "you are what you think." Regardless of who said what, it's been known for centuries that You are What You Eat and What You Think.

The question is, What do You Eat... and What do You Think?

Maybe you're caught somewhere in this 'vicious' cycle of worry and fear, along with a poor diet, and lack of exercise, financial woes, relationship difficulties, lack of spiritual connection, maybe you need to look at what you're feeding your body, mind, and spirit.

Are You caught in this....

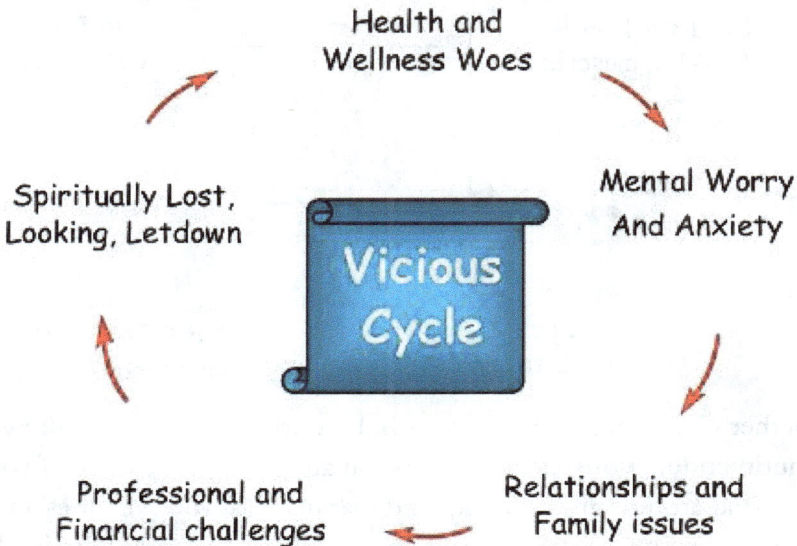

Health and
Wellness Woes

Spiritually Lost,
Looking, Letdown

Vicious
Cycle

Mental Worry
And Anxiety

Professional and
Financial challenges

Relationships and
Family issues

As an adult, whether you realize it or not, **You Are the Chef!**
You're responsible for what you feed your body, mind, and spirit.

You decide how good or bad you want to feed your body, mind, and spirit. Life is all about Choices! You don't have to feed yourself perfectly every day, every meal. But you do want to consume more of the good stuff than bad.

This is what **5 STEPS a Day** is all about. It's helping you move into that 'virtuous' circle by improving your Habits and Attitudes, by tracking how you feed your body, mind, and spirit.

5 S.T.E.P.S. to move into this...

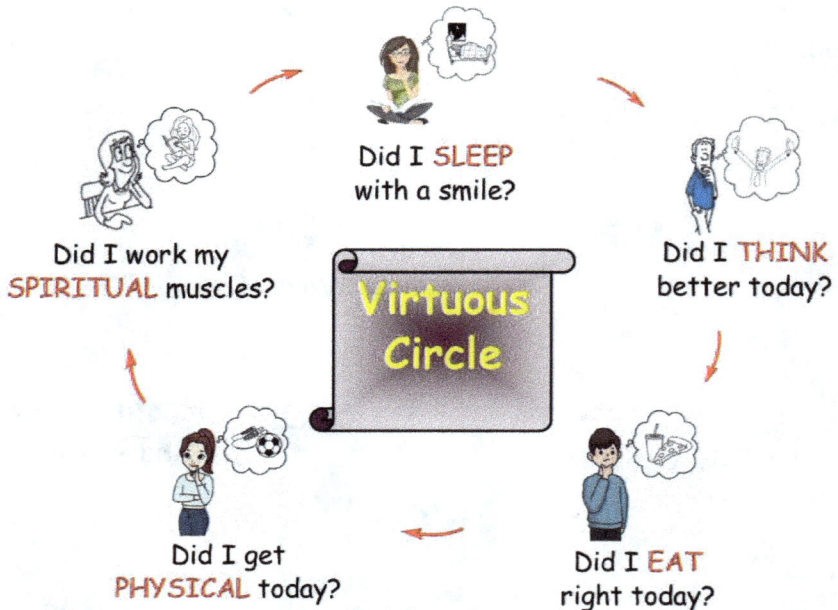

Did I **SLEEP** with a smile?

Did I work my **SPIRITUAL** muscles?

Virtuous Circle

Did I **THINK** better today?

Did I get **PHYSICAL** today?

Did I **EAT** right today?

Whether you realize it or not, **your habits and attitudes are like your genetic code... your DNA** of who you are. Trace back some of your habits and attitude and you may find that many of your victories and accomplishments were a result of your habits and attitude. But by the same token, some of your challenges and difficulties can be traced back to some of your less than desirable habits and attitudes. So, maybe depending on where you are in your life - you may need to CHANGE some of your habits and attitudes?

- *Brushing your teeth, flossing, taking your vitamins are good habits.*

- *Hours of social media, gaming and television aren't so good.*

- *Negative self-talk, doubt, and worry doesn't helping you!*

- *Developing your Self-confidence and Belief in Yourself does!*

Think of your habits and attitudes like an airplane's auto-pilot system. Set the autopilot correctly, and the plane will get you where you want to go, even with the wind in your face. But if your autopilot isn't set correctly, you may be in for a bumpy ride.

Let me say it another way, if you want to CHANGE your circumstance, CHANGE your situation – you are going to have to change some things. You can't keep doing the same thing, hoping for a different result.

CHANGE is not a 4-letter word!

CHANGE doesn't happen by accident!

CHANGE IS INTENTIONAL!

Change is about...

Creating Habits and
Attitudes Now for Greater
Expectations.

"The journey of a thousand miles begins with your first step"

Lao Tzu

Sleep **Think** **Eat** **Physical** **Spirit**

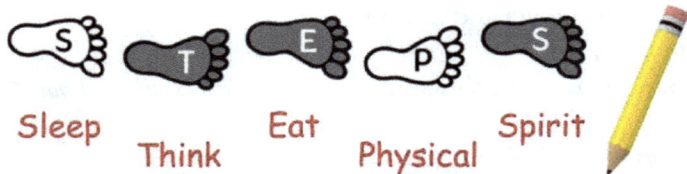

5 STEPS a Day is all about 'readying Your ship to sail.' You may not know exactly where it is you want to go or what you want to achieve tomorrow, next week, next month, or next year. But as you 'ready your ship to sail' by strengthening your body, mind, and spirit. You'll be better equipped to handle the various challenges and difficulties so you can move from that Vicious cycle into that Virtuous circle.

What makes **5 STEPS a Day** different than other accountability journals and to-do lists is that we are tapping into all those Visual and Kinesthetic learners who don't get inspired or motivated by simply reading or listening to another self-help guru.

In less than 2 minutes a day you can quickly track your habits and attitude by shading-in the footsteps of your action.

➢ Did I EAT right today? Shade in the 'E'
➢ Did I get PHYSICAL (exercise) today? Shade in the 'P'
➢ Did I THINK better today? Shade in the 'T'
➢ Did I SLEEP and Dream good thoughts? Shade in the first 'S'
➢ Did I work my SPIRITUAL muscles today? Shade in the last 'S'

You're creating an image... a picture... that you can visually see of all your progress. There's something about visually seeing all your steps... your progress... that taps into your visual and kinesthetic learning centers to help anchor those better habits and attitudes.

·

It's NOT Rocket Science!

It's ACCOUNTABILITY AND FEEDBACK!

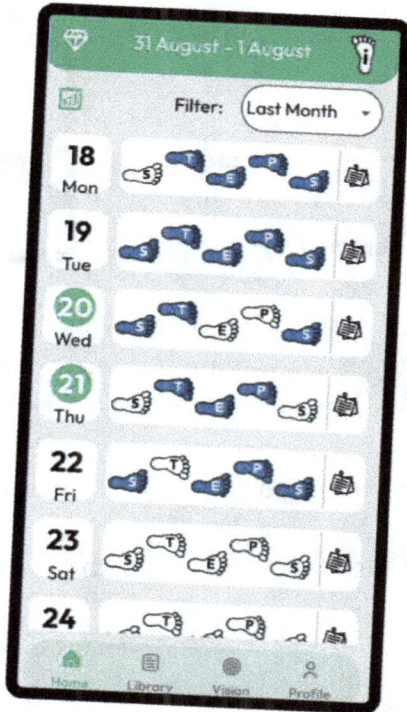

Are you doing the things that are in your DNA that are known to make you Healthy, Wealthy and Wise? Or at least make you **Bigger, Better, Bolder** so you can overcome whatever Giants that are in your path!

There's nothing else like

5 STEPS a Day!

> ✓ Is your level of health and fitness where you want it to be?
> ✓ Are your personal relationships thriving?

> ✓ Are you expanding your professional opportunities?
> ✓ Is your spiritual walk where you want it to be?

Maybe you need to make some changes.

Let me now introduce you to each of the S.T.E.P.S.

Ralph Waldo Emerson said, *"it's the journey – not the destination."*

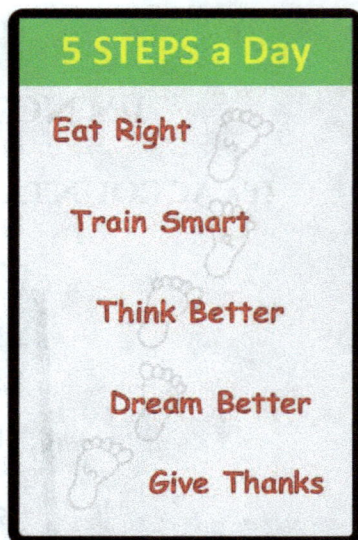

5 STEPS a Day

Eat Right

Train Smart

Think Better

Dream Better

Give Thanks

PHYSICAL

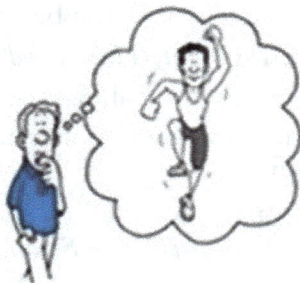

Did I get PHYSICAL today?

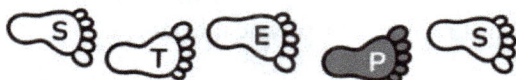

If you did, shade-in the 'P'

Your Body is Your Temple! Does it need a little maintenance work or a complete makeover? I'm not asking if it was a hard or easy workout? If it was aerobic or anaerobic? Or if it was a short or long workout. Did you carve out some time in your day to do some type of physical exercise or activity?

I'm not asking if you did your 10,000 steps or closed your rings? Nor am I asking if you lifted weights, ran, biked, danced, swam, or played pickle ball! Keep in mind, for some people walking to the store, gardening, cutting the grass or shooting hoops with the kids could easily count as physical exercise for the day.

Don't over-analyze the question, did you carve out some time in your day to get some physical activity? Did you take a step forward today or not? If you did, lock in that gratification, get that mini-victory and shadein your step. If you didn't - tomorrow is another day, and you'll have another chance to take a step forward. And don't get down on yourself if you didn't get your regularly scheduled, complete workout in.

Keep in mind, physical exercise may not be one of those things you do every day. It's different than *Eat, Think, and Sleep*... which are things you do every day. The simple goal is to make physical exercise or activities a positive habit for yourself because it impacts both your mental and physical health.

Don't forget the term, '*Strong Body – Strong Mind*' has been around for centuries. Maybe it's the physical exertion that makes you feel strong or stronger about yourself. Or it could be the feeling of achievement and accomplishment from within. Or the endorphin hit you receive when you exert and move your physical body.

Either way, Your Body is Your Temple! You decide how much effort you want to put into your temple. You may want to train like an Olympian or someone who simply wants to **Look Better, Feel Better and Sleep Better**.

EAT

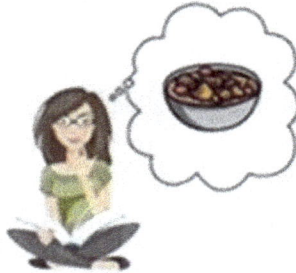

Did I **EAT** right today?

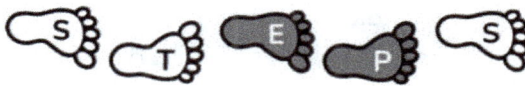

If you did, shade-in the 'E'

Garbage In – Garbage Out! If you are trying to improve your level of health, lose weight, get in better shape or overcome some health issue… Your diet and what you EAT is important! More importantly, you are your own personal chef – for Yourself! So, you get to decide how good, or how bad, you want to feed your body.

Are your dietary choices helping or hindering you? You can't get healthy and trim if you don't Eat right, it's that simple! You don't have to eat perfectly, but you do need to Eat better.

Did you eat good for the day? Did you leave off that second serving, dessert, junk food, sugary snacks, a late-night binge and all the sugary bad drinks for the day? Do you need to change some of your dietary habits? I'm not asking you to count calories, fats, or carbs. Nor am I asking if it was organic or not. Or if you followed your dieting program – perfectly. I'm looking for good meals and better dietary choices for the day, for the week - not perfect meals.Everyone's coming from different starting points regarding our dietary needs and choices. I'm not looking to beat up refined, packaged, or processed foods. Yes, organic, grass fed is better but for some people, simply staying away from that second serving, junk foods, desserts, late-night snacks, soft drinks, and lattes with 5 squirts of sugar... are a big step in the right direction.

If you can eat three good meals a day that's awesome! Shade in your step. Keep in mind, two good meals and one not so good meal is essentially taking two steps forward and one step back. You still made progress! Home runs are great, but base hits will also help you win.

Maybe you splurged or had a decadent meal? OK! Did you keep it to only one bad meal or did you drop the ball for the whole day? The rest of the week? If you did well and had more good meals than bad for the day, pat yourself on the back, shade in your step and keep moving forward.

Unfortunately, for some people, when they screw up and blow a meal, it can sabotage their whole week. So, don't over-analyze your results. You simply want to eat more good meals than bad ones for the day, for the week. And 17 good meals and 4 not so good meals for the week is a lot better than 12 good and 9 bad meals. So, if you did Eat right for the day, **shade-in the E** and pat yourself on the back.

THINK

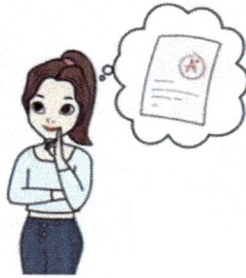

Did I THINK better today?

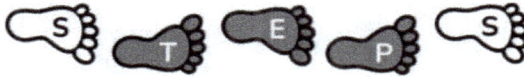

If you did, shade-in the 'T'

You Reap What You Sow! Your mind is always thinking and processing thoughts. It starts from the moment you wake up until the time you go to sleep. The thing you need to remember is that you are the chef who is responsible for choosing what to feed your mind. Do you tell yourself and create a mindset that it's going to be a great day first thing in the morning? Or do you wait till after a shower, after breakfast, walking the dog, feeding the kids, driving to the office, after your workout, etcetera. How long does it take before you give yourself some positive word of encouragement?

Researchers estimate that we process more than 50,000 thoughts a day. They also say that 80% of those 50,000 thoughts are from yesterday. And 90% of yesterday's thoughts are Negative. Another words... more than 80% of your daily thoughts areNegative Re-runs from Yesterday! So, let's get into a better habit of feeding our mind with some better thoughts to chew on.

Positive thinking goes back to biblical times, when we first heard *a man is as a man thinketh.* So, what kind of self-talk are you feeding yourself? Is your internal dialogue telling you *Yes, I Can or No, I Can't?* Are you telling yourself that you're **Bigger, Better, Bolder?** Or do you keep feeding those 'little giants' in your head that tell you that you're Doomed, Dazed and Defeated? Are you building up your self-esteem and confidence or not? You don't need to repeat a magic phrase a bazillion times, but you need to add some positive thoughts and affirmations to your daily mental diet. The last thing you want to do is allow your mind to be filled with thoughts of No, I can't – Not me, Not Today!

Yes, positive self-talk might feel a little awkward in the beginning, but that doesn't mean it's wrong. You need to change your internal dialogue to something that inspires and motivates you, not limits you! It's called **self-talk** and if people can **exercise, dine, travel, shop, and sleep by themselves.** Why can't you talk to yourself and give yourself some positive words of encouragement. It's a lot less expensive than paying for a coach!

It's easy to get **mentally distracted** after you wake up – with all that's going on, but you need to be mindful of your thoughts and your internal dialogue and get it to help you, not hinder you? Take a minute or two after you wake up and give yourself some positive words of encouragement, a mini pep talk. Just remember, the world isn't filled with **born leaders and positive thinkers** – they are learned skills. The question is, are you going to learn and practice these skills or not? It's easy to tell yourself... *work sucks, I can't do it, I can't buy a break, yada, yada, yada.* All I'm trying to do is get you to start adding a few more drops of something positive and uplifting into our mental diet and start moving the scale in the other direction. Remember more than 80% of your thoughts are slanted negatively. And I know some of you are thinking can a one- or two-minute pep talk really help? Let me answer it this way, that one or two-minute pep talk you give yourself – will at least keep you from dogging yourself for one or two minutes.

SLEEP

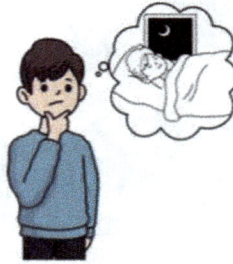

Did I **SLEEP** with good thoughts?

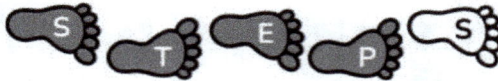

If you did, shade-in the 'S'

Did I **Sleep with a Smile and good thoughts** as I *Dreamed about My Tomorrow?* Or did I fall asleep with thoughts of worry, fear, and anxiety... with my phone in my hand? I'm sure you know it's not good to feed your body junky food before bedtime – so why would you choose to feed your mind junky thoughts before going to sleep?

Did you feed your subconscious with positive, uplifting thoughts, and dreams for tomorrow? Did you know that the thoughts you feed your subconscious will get replayed throughout the night, and can affect your tomorrow?

I'm NOT asking how many hours you slept, or if you fell asleep quickly, or if you woke up and couldn't go back to sleep. But if you go to bed grumpy, anxious, or worried about tomorrow - what kind of attitude or mindset do you wake up with? Whereas, if you fall asleep with a **smileon your face**, as you visualize your goals, dreams, and accomplishments, what kind of attitude and mindset do you wake up with?

Sleeping with a Smile happens when you take those last minutes before falling asleep to focus and visualize your goals, dreams, and aspirations. The more vivid that mental picture in your head, the bigger that smile grows on your face – it's one of those Pavlov's dog things. Simply close your eyes and start visualizing whatever goal, dream, or aspiration you want to see happen. You can dream about something that's 5 years or 5 days from today. What you will notice as the image in your mind gets more vivid and in focus – the bigger and bigger the smile grows on your face. That's what **Sleeping and Dreaming with a Smile is all about!**

I know some people may not know exactly what their goals and dreams are, but that doesn't mean you can't *'ready the ship to sail.'* You can still build up your confidence and self-esteem with simple words or affirmations at bedtime like, *I feel great; tomorrow will be a great day, I'm healthy and strong.* It's your choice, you can fall asleep with the remote or your phone in your hand. Or you can give yourself some direction and purpose and Dare to Dream about what it is you want to achieve or see happening in your life.

You spend a third of your life asleep, under the control of your subconscious. You decide if you want to nourish it with positive or negative thoughts. Keep in mind...

If you can't imagine your dreams coming true with your eyes closed, how in the heck do you expect them to happen with your Eyes Wide Open? Give your mind something to focus on. Give it some direction, a destination! I'm no sailor, but I do know, you don't set sail without knowing where you want to go.

> *If you're not focused on getting to Your proverbial land of milk and honey – don't complain if you arrive in the land of Headaches and Heartaches.*

If Sleeping with a Smile is tapping into the power of your subconscious, doesn't it make sense to have your subconscious mind working for you as opposed to working against you.

A Dream Board (vision board) can be very helpful with your **5 STEPS**.

SPIRIT

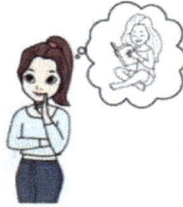

Did I work my **SPIRITUAL** muscles?

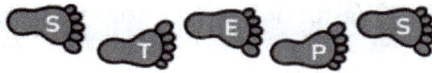

If you did, shade-in the last 'S'

Neglecting Your Spirit is Like Skipping a Meal – It Leaves You Empty! You can't exercise once a week and expect to be physically strong. Nor can you expect to be spiritually strong by only working your spiritual muscles once a week, once a month, or less? The same applies for being born into any religious belief – it doesn't guarantee spiritual strength. You have to invest some time and energy, because you are **Body, Mind,** and **Spirit.**

Similar to your physical muscles, you get out of it what you put into it! And like your physical muscles there are different ways to strengthen your spiritual muscles. I know we all come from different starting points! Some question a higher power. Some were raised with religious beliefs, others weren't, and some were taught it was nonsense. In other words, some of us may be lost, looking, or letdown in our spiritual walk.

For years I had my doubts and have gone full circle. I wasn't connected and growing in my spiritual walk, but I finally started to ask questions.I put in my time and effort to read and learn for myself. And it's true, "when the student is ready, the master will appear."

One thing that was eye opening for me was when I learned that the writings of Aristotle, Socrates, Homer, and Hippocrates, the father of medicine, all lived more than 2,000 years ago. However, we only have a handful of manuscripts that were written hundreds of years after their death... and they are accepted as accurate and true. Yet we have thousands of gospel manuscripts that were written and dated back to the same century as when Jesus walked the land. And we're questioning their validity and authenticity? And hasn't the world been dating TIME as BC (before Christ) and AD (after death) for more than 15 centuries?

Anyway, years ago I realized I was only strengthening my spiritual muscles once a week, if at that. How strong could my spiritual muscles really be? Could I be physically strong if I only exercised my body once a week? No, so I started reading, studying, fellowship with others and this was all before cell phones. But this little device that we all carry with us can connect us with so much information, podcasts, television programs, and music at your fingertips. So, there are so many different ways and opportunities to strengthen your spiritual walk anytime during the day. The question is, are you taking the time or not?

Don't **Neglect your Spiritual Muscles!** There are several different ways you can exercise your spiritual muscles. Let me also say, some people haven't had their spiritual muscles tested – YET. And who's to say that maybe you're meant to be the crutch to help someone else in their time of need.Either way, the simple goal is to strengthen your spiritual muscles more than once a week, once a month, twice a year. Like your physical muscles – you may not need them all the time, but it's great to have them when you do need them.

As I conclude my writing, let me share this poem with you... I won't share the title, see if you can figure it out?

I am your constant companion.

I am your greatest helper or your heaviest burden.

I will push you onward or drag you down to failure.

I am completely at your command.
Half the things you do you might as well turn over to me,
And I will be able to do them quickly and correctly.
I am easily managed; you must merely be firm with me.
Show me exactly how you want something done,
And after a few lessons I will do it automatically.
I am the servant of all great individuals
And, alas, of all failures as well.
Those who are great I have made great
Those who are failures I have made failures.
I am not a machine,
Though I work with all the precision of a machine
Plus the intelligence of a human being.
You may run me for profit or run me for ruin;
It makes no difference to me. Take me, train
me, be firm with me,
And I will put the world at your feet
Be easy with me, and I will destroy you.

Who am I?

I AM HABIT!

Author Unknown

If you keep doing what you've been doing - you'll keep getting what you've been getting. If you want tomorrow to be different from yesterday, you have to do something different today.

Can I guarantee better habits and attitudes will bring health, wealth, and happiness. NO - **but it sure does increase your odds.**

One last thing, the coolest thing about **shading in** your STEPS and **Visually** seeing your progress every day is that you get this little feel good, bio-chemical, endorphin hit for your accomplishment. You don't get that from reading or listening to other self-help programs.

If you prefer paper and pencil, try our **5 STEPS Calendar** or **Journal.** If you prefer an app, there's the **5 STEPS a Day app.**There's also a **TEEN** version. **The STEPS** are the same, but Different. In case you hadn't thought about it. TEENS get complete control of what they put into their 'mental shopping cart' by the start of their second decade. No learners permit or training manual to help manage that internal voice that's always in your ear.

I appreciate your time, good luck on Your Journey.

Dr. Len

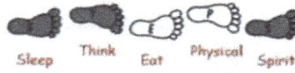

My **5 STEPS**

Sleep   Think   Eat   Physical   Spirit

Calendar

107

NOTES

NOTES

Chapter 9

The Art of Cellular Wellness: A Holistic Approach to Healing By Dr. MaryAnn "Dr. O" Woods Osifo, DC

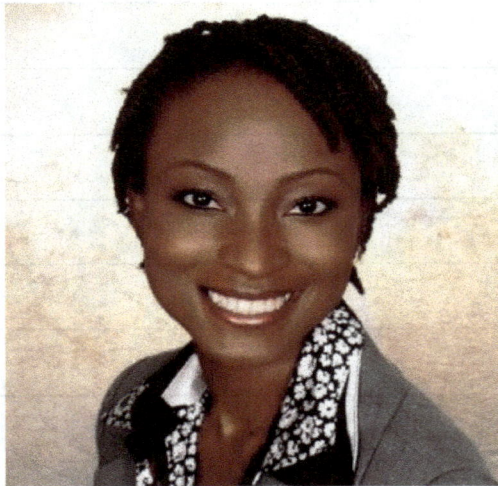

Dr. MaryAnn "Dr. O" Woods-Osifo, DC

Chiropractor · Wellness Advocate · Community Leader

Biography

Dr. MaryAnn Woods-Osifo—affectionately known as "Dr. O"—is a distinguished chiropractor and holistic wellness leader based in McKinney, Texas. Originally from Monrovia, Liberia, her transition from West African roots to North Texas exemplifies resilience, purpose, and the power of healing.

She earned her Doctor of Chiropractic degree from Parker University in 2013 and holds three bachelor's degrees in Biological Science, Human Anatomy, and Health & Wellness. During her academic journey, she was recognized as a Pioneer of Chiropractic by the World Federation of Chiropractic and served as president of the Distinguished Toastmasters Club, among others. Her early scholarly work included co-authoring research on herbal supplement usage among U.S. adolescents.

Practice & Philosophy

In 2024, Dr. O launched Dr. O Chiropractic and Wellness Lifestyle, her signature wellness clinic. She is guided by the principle that the body—when properly supported—possesses a natural ability to heal.

Her offerings span spinal decompression, neuropathy therapy, red-light treatment, and comprehensive wellness planning tailored to individual needs. With over 50,000 treatments administered, Dr. O is a trusted healer and wellness partner in her community.

Recognition & Leadership

Dr. O has been honored twice as Best Chiropractor in McKinney (2016, 2021), a reflection of both clinical excellence and community trust. She is also a sought-after speaker, mentor, and advocate who empowers others to embrace holistic health and wellness.

Dr. O lives in McKinney with her husband and family, continuing her vision of accessible, compassionate care and inspired living.

Connect with Dr. O

- **Website:** drosifo.com

- **Email:** dro@drosifo.com

The Art of Cellular Wellness: A Holistic Approach to Healing
By Dr. MaryAnn Woods-Osifo, DC

About the Author

Dr. MaryAnn Woods-Osifo is a passionate chiropractor specializing in natural, non-invasive therapies. With a deep commitment to holistic health, her approach focuses on long-term wellness, healing from the inside out, and nurturing the body on a cellular level. Her personal journey of resilience, shaped by the loss of loved ones, drives her dedication to helping others achieve physical, emotional, and spiritual well-being.

Dr. Woods-Osifo's path began in Liberia, West Africa, where she was born and raised. In 1990, during the civil war, she and her family left the country to seek new opportunities and safety in the United States. The loss of her brother in 2002 and her father in 2005 ignited a profound desire in her to help others heal, which ultimately led to her dedication to chiropractic care and holistic wellness.

Chapter Overview

The Art of Cellular Wellness delves deep into the essential role that cellular health plays in overall well-being. Through personal experiences, scientific insights, and professional expertise, Dr. Woods-Osifo provides a comprehensive look at how nurturing your cells can transform your health. The chapter explores the intricate connection between cellular health and various aspects of daily life—including nutrition, hydration, exercise, stress management, and sleep—offering practical advice on how to achieve vitality and long-term wellness by starting at the cellular level.

Contents Include

- Dr. MaryAnn's personal journey of healing and resilience

- The importance of cellular health in overall well-being

- The role of mitochondria in energy production and vitality

- Strategies to slow the aging process by supporting cellular health

- Practical guidance on daily habits: nutrition, hydration, exercise, and stress management

- The impact of emotions and mindfulness on cellular regeneration

- Holistic approaches to maintaining long-term vitality and wellness

Contact Information

Dr. MaryAnn Woods-Osifo, DC
dro@drosifo.com
www.drosifo.com

The Beauty of Cellular Health: A Holistic Approach to Recovery

My Story of Strength and Recovery

Reflecting on the journey that led me to a place where I can support others in their healing process brings a sense of gratitude and purpose to my heart. My story traces back to Liberia, West Africa, where I spent my early years. In 1990, my mother, brother, and I left due to the civil war, seeking safety and a fresh start in the United States, full of hope for a brighter future.

Despite our efforts to build a new life, life's struggles remained present. In 2002, my world changed forever when I lost my beloved brother, followed by my father's passing in 2005. Grief, as many of us know, can either shatter you or propel you toward a higher purpose. For me, it served as a driving force—a source of motivation that led me to dedicate myself to the field of healing.

I chose a path of gentle, natural treatments that work in harmony with the body's own healing capacities. Today, my clinic is not just a place for therapy—it's a sanctuary for holistic well-being, where individuals can nurture their physical, emotional, and spiritual growth. Healing from within begins at the cellular level, and I am deeply committed to guiding people on their journey to wellness.

The Importance of Cellular Health

Everything begins with your cells—the tiny building blocks that sustain your existence. Your body is composed of approximately 37 trillion of these microscopic units, each with its own unique role. I like to think of them as performers in a grand symphony, working in perfect harmony to create the melody of your life. From every heartbeat to every thought, your cells are the very essence of vitality and energy.

When your cells are stressed or not functioning optimally, your body feels off. The health of your cells affects every aspect of your well-being—from cognitive function and heart health to your ability to move and breathe. Research emphasizes how intricate and interconnected our cells are, acting as the foundation of human health and well-being (Hatton et al., 2023). When our cells are thriving, we are thriving.

Every cell in our body has a specific role, whether it's protecting us from infection, supporting our muscles as we move, or helping our brain process complex thoughts. When you care for your cells, you're taking care of the foundation upon which your health and life rest. The idea of "cell love" isn't just a figure of speech—it's a practical, meaningful approach to living a full, healthy life.

The Inner Power Source: Embracing Your Mitochondria

Some days you feel like you can conquer the world, while other days even getting out of bed feels like an insurmountable challenge. A lot of this fluctuation comes down to your mitochondria—the tiny powerhouses within your cells that convert the food you eat and the air you breathe into energy.

When your mitochondria are healthy, you feel vibrant, focused, and energetic. But when they're under stress, fatigue sets in. Research by Annesley & Fisher (2019) highlights how mitochondrial dysfunction is linked to chronic fatigue and neurodegenerative conditions.

Nurturing your mitochondria through regular activity, a healthy diet, and stress management is an essential act of self-care. Studies show that habits like walking, cycling, and consuming antioxidant-rich foods can significantly boost mitochondrial function (Garatachea et al., 2015).

Aging Gracefully: Slowing Down the Clock on Your Cells

As we age, cells lose vitality and become more vulnerable to oxidative stress. Fortunately, lifestyle choices can slow this process. Regular physical activity, anti-inflammatory foods, and sleep all help reduce "inflammaging"—a term describing age-related chronic inflammation.

By staying active, eating turmeric, green tea, and leafy greens, and managing stress, we reduce inflammation's impact on our cells and maintain overall well-being.

Nourishing Your Cells with Care

Each meal is an opportunity to fuel your body on a cellular level. Antioxidants protect cells from oxidative damage. Foods like blueberries, spinach, and nuts help your cells function efficiently. Protein and omega-3s help repair and strengthen cell membranes, supporting both brain and immune health.

Hydration: The Purest Form of Love

Water supports every cellular function—from transporting nutrients to flushing toxins. Even mild dehydration impacts cell efficiency (Häussinger, 1996). Stay hydrated with water-rich foods like cucumbers, oranges, and watermelon.

Movement: Energizing Your Cells

Exercise boosts oxygen flow, mitochondrial function, and overall cellular health (Marsh & Coombes, 2005). Movement promotes repair and regeneration, making it a non-negotiable for vitality.

Managing Stress: The Silent Enemy of Your Cells

Chronic stress increases inflammation and accelerates cellular aging. Practices like mindfulness, deep breathing, and meditation reverse this effect, helping your cells regenerate (Valera-Alberni & Canto, 2018).

Sleep: The Ultimate Act of Self-Care

Sleep is when your body repairs and detoxifies. Deep rest supports antioxidant defense and cellular healing (Everson et al., 2005). Prioritize consistent, high-quality sleep for long-term health.

The Science Behind It All: Telomeres, Autophagy & Inflammation

Telomeres are protective caps at the ends of your chromosomes. Each time a cell divides, telomeres shorten. When they become too short, the cell can no longer function properly. Stress, poor diet, and lack of sleep accelerate this shortening. Conversely, exercise, a nutrient-dense diet, and emotional resilience can preserve telomere length—delaying aging and disease (Zgraggen, 2021).

Autophagy is your body's natural recycling system. It allows cells to remove damaged components and reuse valuable parts. Fasting, high-intensity exercise, and deep sleep activate autophagy—making them powerful anti-aging tools.

Inflammation plays a double role. While acute inflammation helps heal injuries, chronic low-grade inflammation silently damages cells. This "inflammaging" has been linked to conditions like diabetes, heart disease, and Alzheimer's. Managing it through anti-inflammatory foods, stress reduction, and cellular hydration is essential for lasting health.

The Cellular Wellness Toolkit

1. **Morning Hydration Ritual:** Start your day with 12–16 oz. of warm lemon water to wake up your cells and flush toxins.

2. **Cell-Loving Nutrition Plan:** Build meals around:

   o Leafy greens

   o Berries (blueberries, raspberries)

   o Healthy fats (avocados, walnuts, flaxseed)

   o Lean proteins (salmon, quinoa)

3. **Movement for Mitochondria:**

   o 30 minutes of moderate activity (walking, dancing, yoga)

   o At least 2 days a week of resistance training

4. **Digital Detox Breaks:** Take 10 minutes daily to unplug, breathe, and reset. Use apps like Insight Timer for guided stress relief.

5. **Sleep Hygiene Setup:**

   o   No screens 1 hour before bed

   o   Magnesium-rich dinner (leafy greens, pumpkin seeds)

   o   Sleep in complete darkness and quiet

6. **Weekly Reset:** One day a week, go plant-based and unplug socially. Let your cells rest and reset.

Daily Practices for Long-Term Cellular Love

Caring for your cells is a lifelong commitment. By making intentional choices—eating well, moving daily, managing stress, and sleeping deeply—you equip your body for vitality at every stage of life.

References

1.   Abd El-Hack, M. E., et al. (2021). *Curcumin and its effects on health.* Journal of the Science of Food and Agriculture.

2.   Annesley, S. J., & Fisher, P. R. (2019). *Mitochondria in health and disease.* Cells, 8(7), 680.

3.   Brod, S., Rattazzi, L., Piras, G., & D'Acquisto, F. (2014). *Emotion and the immune system.* Immunology.

4.   Everson, C. A., Laatsch, C. D., & Hogg, N. (2005). *Antioxidant defense responses to sleep loss.* American Journal of Physiology.

5.   Garatachea, N., et al. (2015). *Exercise attenuates the major hallmarks of aging.* Rejuvenation Research, 18(1), 57–89.

6. Häussinger, D. (1996). *Cellular hydration in cell function.* Biochemical Journal, 313(3), 697–710.

7. Marsh, S. A., & Coombes, J. S. (2005). *Exercise and the endothelial cell.* International Journal of Cardiology, 99(2), 165–169.

8. Valera-Alberni, M., & Canto, C. (2018). *Mitochondrial stress management: A dynamic journey.* Cell Stress.

9. Zgraggen, S. (2021). *Why you should do a metabolic detox.* Peaceful Living Wellness.

NOTES

NOTES

Chapter 10

Enhancing Your Life Through Small Acts of Kindness By Aldo Mancini

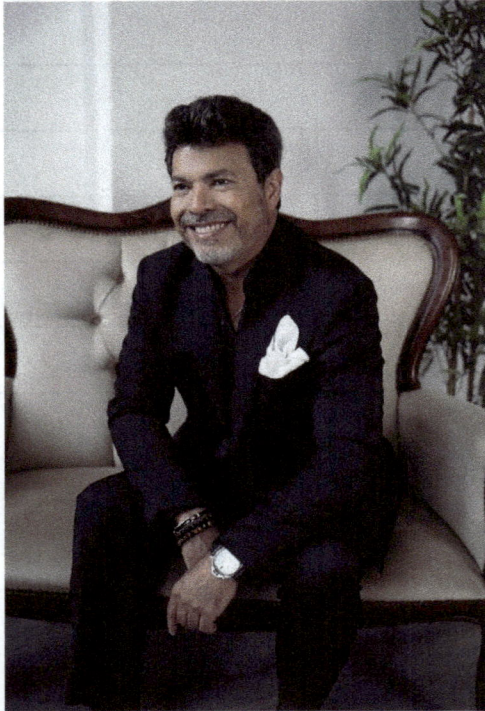

Aldo Mancini is a globally recognized technology executive with leadership roles as Chief Data Officer, Global CIO, and CTO across the Americas, Europe, and Asia Pacific, including companies such as American Express, Discover Financial Services, and AWS, Aldo has guided organizations through large-scale transformation and innovation.

In this book chapter, Aldo draws from his personal and professional journey to explore how small, intentional acts of kindness can radically enhance our lives. Blending science, psychology, and real-world insight, he offers a practical and heartfelt reflection on the power of compassion.

In a world that often feels hurried and disconnected, the transformative power of kindness has never been more essential. Small acts of kindness—simple, intentional gestures that uplift others—have the potential to profoundly enhance not only the lives of those who receive them but also the well-being of those who give. From reducing stress to fostering deeper social connections, kindness is a universal language that bridges divides, nurtures the human spirit, and reminds us of our shared humanity.

In this chapter, we will explore the science behind kindness, the far-reaching ripple effects it creates, and practical ways to weave kindness into the fabric of daily life—ultimately demonstrating how kindness is a natural catalyst for a more fulfilling, meaningful existence.

The Science Behind Kindness and Its Impact on Well-being

Kindness is often considered a moral virtue, but research increasingly shows it is also a practical tool for enhancing mental, emotional, and physical health. Studies, such as the landmark **BIG JOY study** involving nearly 50,000 participants across 200 countries, demonstrate that even micro-acts of kindness—small gestures like offering a compliment or helping a stranger—significantly increase happiness, social connection, and even physical health.

Tracking kind acts alone has measurable effects: the **Counting Kindnesses Intervention** found that participants who simply recorded their kind acts for a week reported higher levels of happiness, gratitude, and purpose. Kindness is not just "nice to have"; it is a vital component of human flourishing.

At a physiological level, kindness triggers a cascade of neurochemical reactions:

- **Oxytocin**, the "love hormone," is released during kind acts, fostering trust, social bonding, and lowering blood pressure.

- **Dopamine** creates the "helper's high," a feeling of pleasure and satisfaction following acts of generosity.

- **Serotonin** stabilizes mood and helps combat symptoms of depression and anxiety.

- **Endorphins**, the body's natural painkillers, are released, reducing physical pain and promoting emotional resilience.

Beyond emotional benefits, kindness also reduces **cortisol**, the primary stress hormone, by up to 30%. It activates the **parasympathetic nervous system**—the body's natural "rest and digest" system—counteracting the chronic stress response that plagues so many in modern life. Moreover, kindness improves **heart rate variability (HRV)**, a marker of physical and emotional resilience, by up to 12%.

In short, kindness is medicine for the mind, body, and soul.

The Ripple Effect of Kindness

One of the most remarkable aspects of kindness is its contagious nature. A single act of kindness can inspire others to pay it forward, creating a ripple effect that extends through communities and across generations.

Research from **Kindness.org** shows that observing acts of kindness often triggers similar behaviors in others, creating positive feedback loops. This phenomenon, called **moral elevation**, produces a warm, uplifting feeling that motivates altruistic behavior. In experimental studies, witnessing kindness increased the likelihood of paying it forward by up to **40%**.

In a world where negativity can often seem louder, kindness offers a quiet, persistent force that gradually transforms individuals, workplaces, and entire communities.

Practical Ways to Incorporate Small Acts of Kindness

Contrary to popular belief, kindness does not require grand gestures or significant resources. It is often the smallest acts, done with great intention, that leave the most lasting impressions. Here are practical, research-backed ways to make kindness a seamless part of daily living:

1. Transform Routine Tasks into Opportunities

Kindness can be woven into everyday routines:

- Offer your seat during your commute.

- Hold the door open at the grocery store.

- Let another driver merge in heavy traffic.

- Greet strangers warmly.

Studies show that small gestures during mundane activities increase overall life satisfaction by up to **15%**.

2. Leverage Creativity to Amplify Kindness

Creativity magnifies kindness:

- Leave handwritten thank-you notes.

- Create uplifting art for community spaces.

- Share real stories of kindness on blogs or social media.

Creative expressions foster deeper emotional resonance and inspire broader acts of compassion.

3. Foster Kindness at Home

Kindness begins at home:

- Establish family rituals around kindness, such as gratitude letters or volunteering.

- Share chores with empathy, offering assistance without being asked.

- Practice active listening, validating each other's emotions.

Families that embed kindness in their dynamics experience higher levels of trust, harmony, and resilience.

4. Extend Kindness to the Environment

Kindness is not limited to human relationships:

- Pick up litter in your community.

- Plant trees or flowers to support local ecosystems.

- Create pollinator-friendly gardens to protect wildlife.

Environmental kindness cultivates a profound sense of connection to the planet and purpose.

5. Cultivate a Kindness Mindset

Kindness is not just an act—it is a way of being:

- Practice **mindful kindness** by giving others your full attention.

- Reframe negative encounters with empathy.

- Celebrate small acts of kindness daily.

By adopting kindness as a mindset, individuals become anchors of positivity in their communities.

Kindness Strengthens Communities and Relationships

Beyond the individual, kindness has the power to build stronger, more resilient communities.

Kindness as a Catalyst for Resilience

During crises like the COVID-19 pandemic, communities that prioritized kindness—through mutual aid networks or acts of neighborly support—recovered faster socially and economically. Research indicates these communities had **20% faster recovery rates**.

Building Inclusive Communities

Kindness bridges divides across cultural, social, and economic lines:

- Learning a neighbor's language.

- Attending multicultural events.

- Advocating for accessibility in public spaces.

These actions foster inclusivity and dismantle barriers to connection.

The Contagious Nature of Kindness

Each act of kindness has a ripple effect:

- 68% of people who receive a kind act "pay it forward."

- Community kindness initiatives dramatically boost empathy and acceptance toward diverse groups.

Kindness is contagious, and each action fuels a cycle of positivity and human connection.

Economic and Health Benefits

Communities that invest in kindness enjoy tangible benefits:

- Boosted local economies through supportive consumer behaviors.

- Lower crime rates and improved public mental health.

- Increased volunteerism and civic engagement.

Kindness is not just good; it is good business and public health strategy.

Leveraging Technology to Amplify Kindness

In our increasingly digital world, technology offers powerful ways to spread kindness:

- **Social Media Campaigns:** Hashtags like #BeKindChallenge inspire global movements.

- **Kindness Apps:** Tools that track good deeds or suggest acts of kindness help maintain consistency.

- **Online Communities:** Virtual spaces for sharing positive stories create global ripple effects.

Technology, when harnessed thoughtfully, can elevate kindness to a global phenomenon.

The Power of Self-Kindness

Often overlooked, **self-kindness** is just as crucial:

- Practice positive affirmations.

- Engage in mindfulness and meditation.

- Allow room for mistakes and personal growth.

Self-compassion strengthens emotional resilience and enables individuals to offer greater kindness to others.

Conclusion: One Small Act at a Time

Kindness is a transformative force that enhances mental health, builds stronger social connections, fosters community resilience, and even stimulates economic growth. Neurochemical evidence shows that kindness is as powerful as many pharmaceutical interventions for mental well-being—and often without the side effects.

As individuals integrate small acts of kindness into daily life—through micro-practices, creativity, environmental stewardship, and digital amplification—they not only enrich their own lives but also contribute to a more compassionate, inclusive world.

Kindness does not require wealth, status, or extraordinary resources. It only requires intention. A smile, a kind word, a moment of attention—these are the building blocks of a better world.

As we navigate the complexities of modern life, let us remember: **The smallest act of kindness is never wasted. It is the seed from which all greatness grows.**

NOTES

NOTES